Leadership
at every level

a practical guide **for managers**

First published 2001 by emap Public Sector Management
Greater London House
Hampstead Road
London
NW1 7EJ

www.hsj.co.uk

ISBN 1-904009-01-8

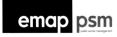

Inside front cover and CD-ROM photo: www.third-avenue.co.uk

CONTENTS

Foreword

Cometh the hour, cometh the manager. Never in its history has the NHS had greater need of effective managers to turn the government's ambitious plans for modernising the service into reality. But today, such is the scale of change, the realisation has dawned that merely to be a manager may not be enough: reform has to permeate so deeply and broadly, it has to reach into the hearts and minds of all the NHS's million staff, that the task calls at every level for *leaders*.

The NHS Executive has noted that, 'Leadership issues continue to dominate the NHS agenda at policy-making, strategic and operational levels.' The service is crying out for leaders to plan for, inspire and motivate its workforce. Acquiring them will involve identifying new leaders and helping existing ones adapt to the new environment. As the NHS plan has it, they should be 'the brightest and the best of public sector management'.

Easier said than done, of course. But a movement is gathering force to enable the NHS to develop the leaders it needs, of which the recently formed NHS Leadership Centre is the figurehead and most obvious symbol. We hope that this practical guide, comprising a book and CD-ROM, will play its part.

As its title suggests, it is intended for health service managers at every level - and from whatever professional background. It eschews the theoretical in favour of providing accessible, easy-to-read support. Leadership may be difficult to define or even describe, but by the time you reach the end of this guide we hope you will have a firm grasp of how qualities of vision, initiative and inspiration distinguish the leader from the manager.

Without doubt, the challenges ahead appear formidable for those seeking to lead the health service. But then the opportunities are immense for anyone equipped to grasp them in order to help re-forge the NHS for the 21st century. And being suitably equipped means feeling at ease with the role of the leader as distinct from that of the manager. The rest is up to you.

Peter Davies
Editor
Health Service Journal

Barbara Harris
Chief Executive
NHS Leadership Centre

October 2001

Acknowledgements

Author

Jeanne Hardacre

Jeanne Hardacre is a fellow at the health services management centre, Birmingham University, undertaking research and consultancy projects in management development, leadership and organisational development. She is a regional tutor for the NHS management training scheme and the programme co-ordinator for the chief executive development programme 'Leading change, delivering the future'.

Editor

Lesley Hallett

Deputy editor, *Health Service Journal*

Editorial Advisors

Professor Jean Faugier

Regional director of nursing, national nurse leadership project

Barbara Harris

Director, NHS Leadership Centre

Dr Peter Lees

Medical director and senior lecturer in neurosurgery, Southampton General Hospital

Karen Lynas

Associate director, NHS Leadership Centre

Additional reseach

Amy Taylor, Linnie Evans

Other acknowledgements

Carol Grant

Partner, Grant Riches Communication Consultants

Carol Ingram

Health services management centre, University of Birmingham

The article *Accountability*, found on the CD-ROM, was originally published on the Wisdom Centre web page, and is reproduced with the Centre's permission (see CD-ROM for further information and a link to the web site).

Getting Teams Started, found on the CD-ROM, is taken from *Exercises for Team Development* by Alison Hardingham and Charlotte Ellis, 1999, with the permission of the publisher, the Chartered Institute of Personnel and Development, CIPD House, Camp Road, London SW 19 4UX.

The creative thinking and problem-solving tools, found on the CD-ROM, are reproduced with the permission of the NHS Clinical Governance Support Team.

Workforce and Development: Embodying leadership in the NHS, found on the CD-ROM, is reproduced with the permission of NHS Executive London.

Design, layout and pictures

Paul Grimes

Rhiannon Frost

"Delivering the plan's radical change programme will require first class leaders at all levels of the NHS."

The NHS plan

Introduction

Leadership — at the heart of modernisation

'Leadership' has become a buzz word within the NHS and there is no doubt that 'leaders' are at the heart of plans to build a modern NHS. *The NHS plan*,[1] published in July 2000, talks frequently of the need for talented and effective leaders in the national health service, and many initiatives have been launched to support the development of leadership skills. (See section on NHS Leadership Centre, page **4**)

It is not easy to describe what leadership is, or to pinpoint what difference it makes to healthcare and health services. Everybody has their own image of what a leader is and how leaders behave, often based on historical or famous characters from the world stage.

Sometimes you instinctively know when you are working alongside a leader, but find it difficult to say what makes you so sure. People viewed as leaders are not necessarily in senior management posts. Very often, leaders are at work on wards and in GP practices, in patients' homes and in hospital laboratories, or behind the scenes supporting those who deal directly with patients.

There has been a good deal of work done by academics, researchers and practitioners to understand what leadership is and to identify what makes a good leader or an effective manager. You will find some reference to this work in the pages that follow, to provide you with some background and context for your role as a leader.

However, this toolkit is not intended to provide comprehensive theoretical information, or to teach you about the theory of leadership. Its main aim is to support you in your working role, to explore your role as a leader, no matter at what level you currently work, and to help you become as effective as possible in your role as leader.

The focus of the toolkit is therefore to provide you with a practical, readable and user-friendly range of ideas, approaches, activities and techniques, designed to help you stretch and develop yourself, explore your further potential and to pursue your own leadership ambitions. The toolkit is of use to anyone who wants to improve their performance.

The approach used throughout this guidebook is not intended to be prescriptive, but rather to raise and discuss key issues and to stimulate new ways of thinking and acting. It offers advice and shares experiences; it provides an extensive source of relevant reading and a range of practical tools.

Working through the guidebook

The CD-ROM

The CD-ROM contains tools such as Internet links, a range of relevant literature and articles, HSJ and a number of tools specially designed by the author to support you in your development as a leader. Further information about the CD-ROM can be found in Appendix A at the back of the book. ➡151

Useful tools

Case histories are drawn from real NHS leaders who have valuable lessons to pass on. Practical and reflective exercises are included throughout the text to reinforce key points. You can carry most of these out on your own, although you may find it useful to consult other members of your team, or your own manager, for some of them.

Symbols

The following symbols are used to guide you to different parts of the text or the CD-ROM:

➡   Activity.

➡   Turn to page.

⟳   Link to CD-ROM.

⌛   See anecdote.

🖱   Link to Internet site.

◆   Internet link cited in book.

This user-friendly working tool offers a great opportunity to develop your leadership skills in your own workplace. And, as the principles of effective leadership are transferable, you will undoubtedly find it a useful working tool to help with the development of other members of your team.

The NHS Leadership Centre

Effective leadership is a key ingredient in changing today's health service. The NHS has some excellent leaders at all levels, but hasn't always supported them with a coherent national programme. Now the new NHS Leadership Centre, part of the Modernisation Agency, is here to support all leaders to realise their potential.

The centre, established in April 2001, brings organisational and personal development together. Many of those working in the centre, including the director, Barbara Harris, come from an operational background that means the work is firmly grounded in reality. Much of the work is about capturing and sharing good practice, to increase effectiveness and drive improvement.

The centre brings together the work of a number of existing teams such as the leadership programme for chief executives, nurse leadership programmes, the management training schemes for general and financial management and the MESOL distance learning programme. There are also pilot programmes for executive directors, doctors, patients and service users' representatives (PALS) and in primary care and mental health.

Since the centre was established, the *Kennedy Report* on the Bristol Royal Infirmary Inquiry has emphasised the importance of this work. It made recommendations about how the centre could support better leadership throughout the NHS. A summary of the centre's response can be found in Appendix B. 153

For more details please visit www.nhs.uk/modernnhs or e-mail us at enquiries@nhs-leaders.org

REFERENCES

1 Department of Health. *The NHS plan - A plan for investment, a plan for reform*, Stationery Office. 2000.

What is leadership?

Introduction

Over the years, there has been a lot of work done to define 'leadership', to understand what leaders do and how they do it, and to uncover the 'secret ingredients' of being an effective leader. This chapter begins with an overview of some of this thinking, providing background and context for your role as a leader. It then discusses the challenges and opportunities of becoming a leader and explores some of the reasons for wanting to develop as a leader and become more effective in your workplace.

Background to leadership

Leadership has traditionally been surrounded by a certain element of mystique, and a view that a leader's ability to achieve great things hinges on a 'charismatic' personality and a talent for inspiring large numbers of people towards a certain goal.

The military provided much of the material for early studies of leadership, and the traits and characteristics of the 'good leader' were the focus of many research studies. These studies explored the idea that leaders were born, not made ('the trait theory of leadership'). However, such research over many years did not result in any consistent and agreed lists of characteristics that could be shown to be innate in successful leaders.

As little conclusive evidence was uncovered about how leadership is influenced by personality, attention switched from studying who leaders are to how they behave. Tannenbaum and Schmidt became closely associated with behavioural theories of leadership. The focus of their research explored how leaders influence the behaviour of others, and was linked to theories of motivation as well as managerial effectiveness. The crux of their work was the differentiation of managers who use high levels of control and authority and those who delegate to others, allowing them freedom to function within defined limits. This work identified two key management styles: 'task-centred' and 'person-centred'. High or low task-centred behaviour can be combined with high or low person-centred behaviour, depending on the circumstances.[1]

Task-centred and person-centred leadership

Task-centred leadership – focuses on tightly controlled planning, organising, monitoring performance and measuring against objectives.

Person-centred leadership – focuses on developing and maintaining relationships, encouraging involvement and participation in decision-making and building mutual trust.

Once some defined management styles had been identified, studies were undertaken to understand which combination of styles was most effective in which circumstances. This led to a range of models that tried to provide a basis for deciding when to adopt which management approach. This work became known as 'situational' or 'contingency' theory, and was significantly shaped by researchers such as Fiedler and Hersey and Blanchard. Professor Fiedler believed that most managers have a personal tendency to adopt a certain style and that the job they do should take account of this.[2] Hersey and Blanchard were of the view that leadership style and the ability to vary this can be developed, and many management development programmes were established on the basis of the situational leadership principle.[3]

Transactional and transformational leadership

Over the past 20 years, a differentiation has developed between 'leadership' and 'management'. Management has become synonymous with 'transactional leadership', which takes place within a hierarchical structure in which the 'leader' has some sort of formal authority over others. This sort of leadership is based on 'position' power, whereby the leader's relationship with others is primarily defined through the nature of the 'transactions' occurring between different levels of authority in an organisation. As such, it may involve an element of coercion or 'pushing'.

Rapid and dramatic developments in the economy in the western world during the 1980s led to awareness that organisations founded on traditional structures were not well placed to respond effectively to rapid and continuous changes. These factors, and an interest in the perceptions of staff on the effectiveness of their leaders led some researchers to identify a different style of leadership, which centred on the ability of the leader to influence others. The term 'transformational leadership' reflects the essence of this style, which is in transforming others' behaviour without recourse to authority or hierarchy. Within this model of leadership, the leader gains and earns their influence from the decision of others to 'follow' or be influenced. Warren Bennis and Kouzes and Posner have been prominent writers in this field.

See CD-ROM for HSJ article 'Maiden over?'

Leadership or management?

'To survive in the twenty-first century we're going to need a new generation of leaders, not managers.'

Warren Bennis[4]

Management has become associated with the characteristics of the 'transactional' model. Leadership is increasingly viewed as having the 'transformational' model at its heart. As the terms 'management' and 'leadership' are often used interchangeably, it can be difficult to know what each really means – and to know whether you want to be a manager or leader, or both. The work of Warren Bennis, a management researcher and academic, helps to clarify this conundrum by differentiating management and leadership, as outlined in the box 'Manager or leader?' below.

A criticism of differentiating management and leadership has been that it implies one is better or more desirable than the other. John Kotter has developed a comparison of how the 'transactional' and 'transformational' approaches contribute to leadership. This demonstrates that elements of both approaches are highly relevant and necessary.

Manager or leader?

- The manager administers; the leader innovates.
- The manager is a copy; the leader is an original.
- The manager maintains; the leader develops.
- The manager focuses on systems and structure; the leader focuses on people.
- The manager relies on control; the leader inspires trust.
- The manager has a short-range view; the leader has a long-range perspective.
- The manager asks how and when; the leader asks what and why.
- The manager has an eye on the bottom line; the leader has an eye on the horizon.
- The manager accepts the status quo; the leader challenges it.
- The manager is the classic good soldier; the leader is their own person.
- The manager does things right; the leader does the right thing.

Warren Bennis, 1985[13]

	Transactional leadership (management)	Transformational leadership (transformational)
Creating the agenda	*Planning and budgeting:* Developing a detailed plan of how to achieve the results.	*Establishing direction:* Developing a vision that describes a future state along with a strategy for getting there.
Developing HR	*Organising and staffing:* Which individual best fits each job and what part of the plan fits each individual.	*Aligning people:* A major communication challenge, getting people to understand and believe the vision.
Execution	*Controlling and problem-solving:* Monitoring results; identifying deviations from the plan and solving the problems.	*Motivating and inspiring:* Satisfying basic human needs for achievement, belonging, recognition, self-esteem, a sense of control.
Outcomes	Produces a degree of predictability and order.	Produces changes – often to a dramatic degree.

Source: JA Kotter, 1990[5]

Activity 1

Think of someone you view as a leader in your organisation and list their key activities/approaches under the heading below which seems to fit best. Then repeat the exercise for yourself in your leadership or management role. How much of a balance is there between transactional and transformational leadership in your organisation?

Transactional	**Transformational**

Leaders and followers

'The leader who looks around and sees only followers will surely fail as a transforming leader.'

Professor Paul Bate [6]

The earlier and more traditional models of leadership are all based on an implicit understanding that leaders 'lead' and followers 'follow' – this certainly seems logical.

However, in the words of Beverly Alimo-Metcalfe, the word 'followers' implies 'passive recipients of the leadership process'.[7] In contrast, embedded in the characteristics of the transformational leader is an emphasis on others taking responsibility, challenging the way things are done, innovating and exploring their potential.

These are not the behaviours of passive followers, and many writers have suggested that a transformational leader's behaviour is more in the mould of 'serving' those around him or her, by creating an environment in which they can thrive and excel in their own right. There is an appreciation that the leader cannot act

alone, underlined by John Heider's view that 'enlightened leadership is service, not selfishness'.[8] Peter Drucker reinforces this point with his observation that leaders tend to talk of 'we' rather than 'I'.[9]

See the CD-ROM for the HSJ article – 'Heaven can wait?' by Beverley Alimo-Metcalfe

Leading modernisation in the NHS

Most leadership writers, researchers and practitioners believe that both transactional and transformational styles of leadership are needed within organisations. It is probably true to say that due to the hierarchical nature of the NHS and many of the health professions (which are now changing), the transactional, management-oriented style has dominated most NHS organisations. Within the newly emerging health organisations, for example in primary care trusts and in health partnership arrangements, there is an opportunity and indeed an important need to decide how leadership in all its forms can best contribute to a modern NHS.

Since the launch of *The NHS plan* in July 2000, plans and initiatives to modernise the health service have all been strongly underpinned by the assertion that effective leadership at all levels in an organisation is one of the keys to successful service improvement. This can be seen by the creation of the NHS Leadership Centre within the NHS Modernisation Agency.

The modernisation agenda within the NHS and in other public sector services is based on changing the NHS from a traditional, hierarchical institution to a responsive service that continually adapts to the need and demands of the environment – most especially its customers, the patients. When considering the development of leadership theory and research over the past few decades, it becomes clear that transformational leadership has a central part to play in this transition. Whilst transactional approaches are still essential to ensure that 'the job gets done', it will be the transformational elements of leadership which will create innovative, modern and forward-thinking approaches to improving health. The most effective leaders are likely to be those who can adopt an appropriate and flexible blend of leadership styles and behaviours.

The NHS plan makes it clear that the biggest challenge facing leaders is to 'redesign' the NHS by putting the patient at its heart and being more responsive to their needs. It will be the job of leaders to influence changes in culture, unite the various staff 'tribes' and

Photo: EMAP Healthcare Open Learning/Richard Smith

Work on leadership is moving away from focusing exclusively on a single individual or manager being the leader.

thus deliver a 21st century service rather than one rooted in the first half of the 20th century.

Leadership behaviours in the NHS

Research work undertaken in the NHS in London has sought to investigate and describe what leadership means in a modernised NHS. This work, entitled *Embodying leadership in the NHS* can be found on the CD-ROM.[10] Based on the views of a wide range of leaders and professionals in the NHS, it describes nine themes of leadership. It then identifies what these themes mean by providing examples under each theme heading of 'What do good leaders do?' and 'What does this mean in practice?'

The nine themes of leadership for modernisation in the NHS are:

1. Articulating the vision
Communicating a broad vision for the whole health community.

2. Motivation
Understanding the need to have a highly motivated organisation.

3. Decision-taking
Being dynamic and proactive in identifying decisions that need to be taken.

4. Releasing talent
Demonstrating the belief that the people within the organisation are individuals with many talents and potential.

5. Responsiveness and flexibility
Valuing flexibility and responsiveness in the organisation.

6. Embodying values
Having a clear sense of personal values.

7. Innovation and creativity
Demonstrating that innovation and creativity are highly valued in the organisation.

8. Working across boundaries
Demonstrating ability to work across professional, team and organisational boundaries.

9. Personal resources
Demonstrating resilience and the ability to call upon reserves of energy.

See CD-ROM for the document 'Embodying leadership in the NHS'

Leaders at every level

If the way in which health services are provided is to be transformed, it is first necessary to transform the way in which organisations work. That means transforming the way things are done, which will have implications on a day-to-day basis for most people. It may mean assessing whether things are being done in the most appropriate way or whether there is a better way of doing them. Openness to continual learning, constant evaluation and development are likely to be pre-requisites of practitioners and managers in responding to the needs and demands of patients and the public.

Activity 2

The NHS plan describes many developments in all areas of the health service that will be needed to bring about the transformation of the NHS. Who do you think is best placed to make these changes into reality? Jot down the names of the people you believe to be key to the process. Do you see these people as 'leaders'?

This activity might raise more questions in your mind than it answers. Perhaps you have identified just one or two people, possibly those who are in management roles, and whom you might expect would be responsible for implementing change. On the other hand, you might have a list of people who provide services more directly, and believe that they are the people who will ultimately determine whether the transformation of services makes a difference to patients.

Increasingly, work on leadership is moving away from focusing exclusively on a single individual or manager being the leader. Rather than thinking about how the 'person at the top' or the 'person in a certain role' can lead everyone else, the key to leadership in a modern context is to consider how all individuals in an organisation can contribute their share of leadership in their own way. Referring back to the transformational model of leadership, this asserts that 'transforming leaders' are those who encourage others to lead. So your level in the organisation does not determine whether or not you are a leader. What is much more significant is how you behave, how others view you, and the way in which you inspire them to want to lead themselves. **9**

Activity 3

Ask yourself: 'Who are the leaders in my organisation? Why do I think this?'

Write down the names that come to mind. Try to decide why you view these people as leaders.

Transition from 'practitioner' to 'leader'

Most people have an area of work in which they have developed experience and skills and so view it as their main focus. They may consider this an area of expertise. People make choices during their careers, which might broaden personal areas of work activity (eg – by taking on responsibility for a larger job). Alternatively, some choose to focus their skills more deeply into a specific area of work (eg – by doing further training in a specialist area of work).

As your experience grows and your skills are developed within the job, you can find yourself faced with decisions about how you want your career to progress. It may be that you reach a point where your current role no longer seems to stretch your capabilities, and it feels time to take on a new challenge. Or

perhaps an opportunity for promotion arises, which seems like the natural next step. Within many professions, there is a clear grading structure, whereby moving up the grades can be seen as making career progress.

It is important to remember that being at a certain grade or level of seniority does not automatically mean that a person is a leader. Different people interpret and perform the same job in a variety of ways, shaping the role with their personality and individual style. Although a more senior role brings with it extra responsibility (and sometimes a better salary), the extent to which that job becomes a leadership role mostly depends on the individual post-holder.

In the same way, leaders can often be spotted in junior roles within an organisation. Whilst

Activity 4

Think of one or two people at work who are in relatively junior roles, but who seem to you to have leadership qualities.

What is it about this person that makes you view them as a leader?

they are not necessarily senior in hierarchical or grading terms, the way they carry out their work demonstrates their leadership skills and potential.

The general leader in mental health services

 I worked as a senior occupational therapist in a community mental health team and then as a team co-ordinator. It was a huge learning curve for me to take on the responsibility of my current job – a large budget, dealing with some difficult staff and having line management responsibility for consultants.

Being a leader in today's NHS is a tremendous challenge, partly due to the tensions between the diverse groups of stakeholders, staff, service users and carers, the local community, political pressures and economic and sociological factors. As a manager and leader, I have to keep abreast of all these issues as well as ensuring that relationships are constantly built and maintained with all groups who have a part to play in the delivery and improvement of care.

The positives about being a leader are the ability to change services and be creative. Change can be disconcerting but it can also be a very liberating experience. If you accept that change will always occur and is a natural feature of the NHS then the best way to deal with it is to become a part of it. By doing so you start to influence change.

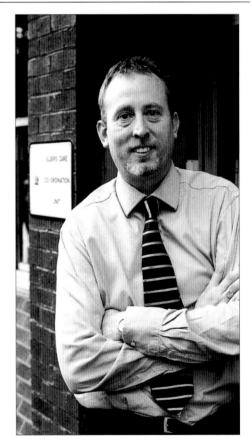

Peter Raimes, East sector mental health service manager, Brent, Kensington and Chelsea Mental Health NHS trust

Photo: Paul Grimes

The senior nursing leader

In my experience, the main challenges involved in moving from the role of practitioner to that of leader was the fact that I no longer belonged to a clearly identifiable 'tribe'. Whilst I had been within the nursing and health visiting community, it was clear who my colleagues and allegiance should be attached to. Once moving out of this close circle, to become a manager, I felt extremely isolated.

It took a while to settle into having to be the one who took the decisions, without necessarily a complete set of information, against competing demands and priorities and extremely tight time scales.

The positive things that I have found about being in a leadership role is the ability to make decisions and shape an organisation or a professional group in the way that you feel is most appropriate. The other most positive area that I have experienced is the ability to nurture and develop junior staff within the health service and to provide them with the opportunity to gain experience and exposure to situations that may not have been available to them previously.

The overriding factor that motivates me in my day-to-day work is the genuine belief that I can make a difference both to the patients and staff within my organisation. I continually strive to meet the targets and deadlines set for us centrally, whilst trying to maintain the balance of ensuring that local issues are dealt with. We must never lose sight of the fact that patients must be our prime focus of attention.

Gill Heaton, director of nursing and operational services, North Cheshire Hospitals NHS trust

The clinical leader

As a trainee in public health, most of my activity was project-based, taking a specific area, examining services, needs and the evidence-base in detail. I naively thought decisions were based on such things.

As a consultant, the pace of life has quickened. I recognise that evidence is not always foremost in determining the direction of change. I realise that the real drivers are much more wide-ranging, multi-faceted and sometimes nebulous. I have surprised myself at my desire to dive into the political, relational and managerial battlefield, but know that my negotiating and influencing skills need to be improved. If I really want to influence thinking and drive change, I still need to develop more confidence and assertiveness.

Rona Cruickshank, consultant in public health

As the case studies in the previous boxes illustrate, these individuals have developed into leaders in their own areas. One has a specialist focus on public health, one has adopted a generalist leadership role and the third has a role combining both clinical and general leadership. Some of the difficulties they have experienced during this transition include:

Shifts from:	▶▶ To:
● Clear understanding of role	▶▶ Interpretation of role
● Reliance on others	▶▶ Self-reliance
● Certainty	▶▶ Ambiguity
● 'Black and white' issues	▶▶ 'All shades of grey'
● A narrow, specialist view	▶▶ A broad overview
● Informing others	▶▶ Persuading/ influencing others

The motivation to lead

In the case studies shown here, the leaders talk about what motivates them in their work. They mention a range of factors, including the desire to improve things and influence others. Of course, leaders are motivated by many different things, depending on their personality, background, experience, outlook on life and their personal values. See pages 17 and 18. **17**

The difference between a clinical or specialist leader and a general leader can be important when identifying your motivation to lead. Clinical leaders are generally people whose main interest is in improving and developing a particular clinical aspect of the patient experience. Their area of focus may cross several different departments or activities. As well as being a practitioner in that area of clinical work, clinical leaders tend to be at the vanguard of innovative approaches and new techniques, keeping abreast of clinical developments and scanning the horizon to anticipate how their clinical area of interest will need to develop in the future.

Clinical leaders are needed in all specialties, across all professions and at all levels. Recent policy initiatives such as the establishment of modern matron, nurse consultants and consultant therapists are all an acknowledgement that clinical leaders will be at the heart of developing a modern healthcare system.

Leaders of a more general nature are also essential to shaping and delivering the modernisation agenda. General leaders are people who have a broader focus on improving the way the whole organisation or an aspect of the organisation works. This is likely to cut across many clinical and non-clinical areas of work. General leaders may have a background in clinical or non-clinical work. They take a lead in understanding changes that will affect an organisation, setting a vision and direction for the future and enabling the way forward.

Clinical and general leaders complement each other and their work is interdependent. The key elements of leadership behaviour identified earlier in this chapter are pertinent to both types of leader, as is the remainder of this toolkit.

Motivation of public sector managers

The Public Management Foundation recently conducted a survey of 400 senior managers (150 public sector, 150 private sector and 100 voluntary sector) about their goals; their sources of job satisfaction; the factors that helped them achieve their goals; and about what their organisations valued. The report concludes that public sector managers are motivated by very different things to their private sector counterparts.

Public sector managers say they are motivated by a desire to produce public value: that is, to benefit service users and local communities. This desire to make a social difference is found right across the sector – in local government, the health service and the police – and at all levels from front-line services to administrative and support functions. Private sector managers' main focus by contrast is on their company's prosperity and performance targets.

Source: *Wasted Values*, Jane Steele, Public Management Foundation

A link to the PMF website can be found on the CD-ROM

As a leader, it is important to be aware of what motivates both you and others. Many interpersonal conflicts and difficulties at work can be due to making incorrect assumptions about other people's reasons for doing things. You will often interpret the behaviour of others using your own set of personal values and motivation tools, and only by appreciating the way other people see things can you gain a real understanding of why they behave the way they do.

For a more detailed and scientific analysis of your motivators, it may be helpful to complete a psychometric instrument such as the SHL motivation questionnaire or the occupational personality questionnaire. Both these must be administered by an appropriately trained person, but you may find that there are people in your organisation who are qualified to do so (possibly in your HR department).

The 'values and motivation at work' questionnaire is a tool to help you define what is important to you at work. This and a link to the SHL website can be found on the CD-ROM

Career anchors

Developing yourself as a leader may form part of your career and development plans. In considering your career moves, it can be helpful to identify those things in your work which are most important to you, and those which may be less crucial.

Edgar Schein developed the idea of 'career anchors'. A career anchor looks at what you perceive to be your skills and talents, your basic values and the motives and needs relevant to your career. Together, these define the things that you want most out of a career, or in Schein's words: 'The career anchor is that one element in a person's self concept that he or she will not give up, even in the face of difficult choices. People typically manage to fulfill a broad range of needs in any given career, but those needs are not all equally important. If all needs cannot be met, it is important to know which ones have highest priority.' [11]

The main anchor categories identified by Schein are:

- Technical/functional competence
- General managerial competence

- Autonomy/independence
- Security/stability
- Entrepreneurial creativity
- Service/dedication to a cause
- Pure challenge
- Lifestyle

Most people are unaware of their career anchors until they are forced to make choices about personal development, career or family. Identifying your career anchors helps you to define those things you are more/less likely to give up, and which will shape the career decisions you make. No matter what your present job or career path, using career anchors can help make future decisions easier and more valid by understanding what is most important to you in your career.

More information about career anchors and career development is provided in the Further reading section on page 143.

Activity 5

A nightmare job

If a job were designed to make your life miserable, what would it be like? Write down the sort of activities you would be doing, where you would be working and with whom you would be.

A perfect job

Design for yourself your most perfect job. Create your own hours, your own activities and decide where and with whom you would work. Allow your imagination to be free, but make sure it is a realistic job, and not just a description of a desirable lifestyle.

Your two lists will tell you a lot about what is important to you in your working life. It is likely that your current job lies somewhere between the 'nightmare' and 'perfection'. Consider how you approach your current job. What are the tell-tale signs that show which parts of the job you like and which parts you don't like?

It is always important to remember that other people will have very different ideas about what is a 'nightmare' or a 'perfect' job. As a leader, if you understand what is important to other people, then you have a better chance of understanding what motivates them to give of their best.

Source: Sher and Smith, 1994 [12]

Embodying values: Having a clear sense of personal values

Personal values have been identified as being a key theme in the way effective leaders in the NHS behave.

What do good leaders do?

Leaders are clear about the values they hold. By demonstrating their values in their day-to-day actions, they persuade rather than impose their values on others. They view excellence in leadership in a positive light, and as a lynchpin of commitment to public sector values.

Leaders demonstrate their personal integrity and command the respect of the people with whom they work. They also show respect for others. In doing so, they behave consistently, although with the flexibility to adapt to particular situations and circumstances. Leaders demonstrate a high level of fairness and justice in their dealings with people but recognise this does not always mean treating everyone exactly the same. They demonstrate a determination to behave equitably, ensuring that all service users have equal access to the services which they need. Leaders also behave equitably in their relationships with staff and colleagues and ensure equal access to opportunities. Leaders acknowledge that values and convictions are best conveyed by personal example.

What does this mean in practice?

- Consistently acting out values in their day-to-day behaviours.

- Demonstrating their respect for the people with whom they work.

- Demonstrating their respect for service users and members of the public.

- Demonstrating fairness and justice in their dealings with people.

- Ensuring equity of access to services for members of the community.

- Ensuring equity of access to opportunities for members of the organisation.

- Demonstrating, in their personal behaviours, high standards of conduct.

- Ensuring that others in leadership roles in their organisation demonstrate the organisation's commitment to fairness, justice, equity and high standards of personal conduct.

Source: *Workforce and Development: Embodying leadership in the NHS*, 2000[10]

Activity 6

Consider each bullet point in turn from the embodying values list opposite. Jot down a recent occasion at work when you behaved in the way described. Try to recall as much detail as possible about the example (eg – who? when? where?)

Do the same again, this time recalling occasions when you know your behaviour did not fit the descriptions given. Again, think through what happened, who was there, etc.

To what extent does your usual behaviour at work fit with the way an effective leader is described here? What can you do to demonstrate your personal values more in your work?

REFERENCES

1 Tannenbaum R, Schmidt WH. How to choose a leadership pattern. *Harvard Business Review* 36/2, 1958: 95-101.

2 Fiedler F. *A theory of leadership effectiveness.* New York; McGraw-Hill, 1967.

3 Hersey P, Blanchard, KH. *Management of organisational behaviour: utilising human resources.* New Jersey; Prentice Hall Inc, 1977.

4 Bennis W. *Managing the dream: Reflections on leadership and change.* Perseus Books, 2000.

5 Kotter JA. *A force for change: How leadership differs from management.* London; Free Press, 1990.

6 Bate SP. Leading the NHS from a different place *Health Services Management Centre Newsletter,* Vol 6 Issue 2, University of Birmingham, 2000.

7 Alimo-Metcalfe B. *Effective leadership.* Local Government Management Board, 1998.

8 Heider J. *The Tao of leadership.* Aldershot; Wildwood House, 1986.

9 Drucker P F. *Management challenges for the 21ˢᵗ Century.* Butterworth-Heinemann, 1999.

10 Workforce and Development Leadership Working Group. *Workforce and development: Embodying leadership in the NHS.* London; NHS Executive, 2000.

11 Schein E H. *Career anchors: Discovering your real values.* Jossey-Bass Pfeiffer Career Series, 1993.

12 Sher B, Smith, B. *I could do anything if only I knew what it was.* Delacorte Press, 1994.

13 Bennis W, Nanus B. *Leaders: The strategies for taking charge.* New York; Harper & Row, 1985.

Notes

> "The quality of leadership, more than any other single factor, determines the success or failure of an organisation."
>
> **Fred Fiedler and Martin Chemers**

Leadership in context

Introduction

Your role as a leader and the development of your leadership skills both contribute to the wide and complex environment in which you operate. An awareness of this environment and how it works is vital, as it allows you to make sense of the complexities and helps you to identify where you fit in.

This chapter provides an insight into the leadership context within your organisation and beyond, and considers how you can develop your awareness, understanding and involvement in this wider leadership environment.

Where your organisation fits in

If you think of your organisation as a complex jigsaw, your service or clinical area represents just one or a few pieces of the whole picture. In order to put your area and your role into context, you need to know what the other pieces of the jigsaw look like. This is why it is useful to learn exactly what services your organisation provides, what other departments exist and to know where they are physically situated. Some of the suggestions in the box on page 29 will enhance your understanding of the services provided by your organisation. **29**

Activity 1

Set yourself the task of learning about every part of your organisational jigsaw – what it is called, where it is located and what service it provides. For example, are there corridors you have never been down - which services are based there? Are there other buildings on or off site or premises where services are delivered – do you know what they are and where they fit into the organisation? Generally, people are flattered if you take an interest in what they do, so don't be afraid to ask.

As well as getting to know more about your own organisation, find out about the key 'partner' organisations in your local community. 'Partner' organisations may include NHS bodies such as acute trusts and primary care groups/trusts etc, GPs, local authorities comprising housing services, social services, education, voluntary organisations, charities, user groups, clinical networks etc. Now try activity 2 on page 28. **28**

Management in your organisation

In Chapter one, you considered whom you view as the leaders in your organisation and what you have noticed about the way they lead. It is possible that some of the people you consider leaders are not in recognised 'management' positions. This emphasises the point that leaders are not always managers, just as managers are not always leaders.

Although managers are not always leaders, it is important to be aware of the formal management structure within your organisation. It is true to say that management hierarchy is less important in some areas of the NHS than it was in the past, eg – in PCTs,

Activity 2

Write the name of your organisation in the middle of the circle below. At the end of each of the lines, write the name of each 'partner' organisation you can think of. Add more lines if you need more. Under each of the partner organisations, write the name of a contact person whom you know in that organisation.

If there are 'partner' organisations for which you do not have a contact name, find one out. If there are 'partner' organisations you do not know very much about, get in touch with them and ask them to send you some general information.

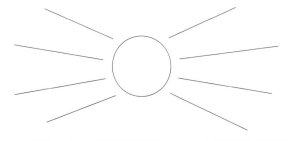

where new approaches to management and leadership are developing. However, in most health-related organisations, the management structure still plays a key role in determining how things are done. As this is likely to have some sort of impact on your own role, it is worthwhile developing an understanding of what the management structure is and whom it comprises.

More details can be found in the HSJ article 'King-Pin Wizards' on the CD-ROM

In order to build an awareness of the management processes in your organisation, you can begin by ensuring that the answers to the questions in the activity 3 on page 30 are 'yes'. Once you have developed an awareness of the managers who impact directly on your area of the organisation, you can follow the same process for managers in other service areas and other specialties. For example, support functions such as human resources and finance impact on all services, so find out about who manages these departments. 30

Learning about how your organisation works

- If you are not clear, ask your manager to help you understand the management structure and decision-making processes in the organisation. You may decide to make this part of your personal development plan.

- Take any opportunities to deputise for your manager at meetings you would not normally attend. There is no reason to feel intimidated or worried about going to such meetings; if on the first occasion you decide to listen and then report back to your manager or team, this is an important contribution in itself.

- Read literature about your organisation, eg – annual report, newsletters, intranet website, and identify the items that affect your service area. Look for names of managers or staff whom you know and note what projects they are involved with.

- Attend an open board meeting. This is the forum, held once a month, where the top management team meets to discuss and agree key issues affecting the organisation. These meetings are open to all staff and the public, so you can just turn up.

- If you are not able to attend, telephone the chief executive's secretary and request a copy of the agenda for the meeting, supporting papers and any minutes of previous meetings. When you receive them, scan these for items affecting your service area to develop your awareness of what is being discussed at senior levels.

- Get hold of a copy of your organisation's strategic plan or annual service plan. Look at what is says about your service area, and if there are things you are not aware of, ask your manager for more information. Bear in mind that he or she may not always be aware of the issues either, so you may need to make your request sensitively.

- Tell your manager that you are interested in understanding more about how your organisation works, and let them know what you are doing to find out, so that this does not come as a surprise to them. If your manager is aware of your interest, he or she may involve you more in broader issues.

- Feed back to your team any information you find out which you think it would be useful for them to know about. Remember you can help others to learn about leadership at the same time as developing yourself as a leader.

→

Activity 3

Get hold of a copy of the organisational chart for your organisation. This is likely to be available from your manager or from the chief executive's office. On the chart, identify where your service area or department sits. Trace the chart down from the chief executive to your own part of the organisation, highlighting the names of all the people in the management structure between you and the chief executive.

The names you have highlighted all play a key role in determining the way things are done in your service area. For each highlighted name, ask yourself:

- Do I know what this person looks like?

- Do I know where this person's office is?

- Do I know anything about this person or their job?

It can sometimes be difficult to know how your department is affected by the senior management in your organisation, especially if you do not have day-to-day contact with senior managers. The box on learning about how your organisation works suggests some ways in which you can gain an awareness of how senior management decisions affect the area you work in. (See page 29)

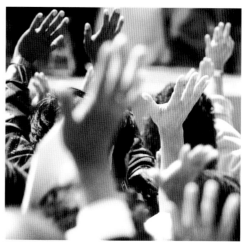

All staff who take decisions about the use of resources contribute to the accountability process.

Accountability and governance

'Who is accountable when healthcare fails? Whom do you blame when your relatives receive sub-standard care? From whom do you seek compensation when you are treated carelessly?'
        'Accountability' by Alan O'Rourke [1]

Leaders in the public sector are responsible for spending public money, and for making sure that this is used to deliver services and improve health in the best possible way. The chief executive of a public sector organisation is ultimately accountable for the financial performance of the organisation, but all staff within that organisation who take decisions about the use of resources contribute to this accountability process. This is likely to include you and the decisions you make.

Activity 4

Talk to your manager about the budget for your service or clinical area. It can be useful to compare it with a domestic housekeeping budget. The following questions may help:

- Who determines how much there is?

- Who decides what the budget should be spent on and how is this decided?

- What are the biggest items of expenditure?

- What happens if there is money left over at the end of the month or year?

- What happens if the budget overspends?

Managers in the public sector are accountable to the public via parliament and the government. The financial accountability of NHS managers has been established for many years, but more recently chief executives of

NHS organisations have also become ultimately accountable for the quality of clinical care delivered under the auspices of their organisation. This new and highly significant level of accountability, known as 'clinical governance', was introduced in the Health Act of 1999. *A First Class Service: Quality in the new NHS* describes clinical governance as: 'a framework through which NHS organisations are accountable for continuously improving the quality of their services and safeguarding high standards of care by creating an environment in which excellence in clinical care will flourish'.[2]

The full version of 'Accountability' can be found on the CD-ROM

Activity 5

Find out how your organisation has responded to the requirements of clinical governance. There are likely to be individuals who take a lead on clinical governance – find out who they are and arrange to talk to them. What impact has clinical governance had in your service area?

Leadership and clinical governance

The Commission for Health Improvement monitors the quality of patient care in NHS organisations by undertaking reviews into how clinical governance is working. Leadership in the organisation is an important aspect considered in the reviews. The following extract from a recent CHI report into an English NHS trust emphasises how important leadership can be in ensuring that services for patients are improved:

'CHI found commitment, enthusiasm and strong leadership for clinical governance at a strategic level. The trust has a strategy for clinical governance but the evident leadership, and the commitment of staff, is not matched by an articulated vision of how the process will lead to the improvement of services for patients. Without such an articulated vision it may be difficult for the trust, and its patients, to appreciate just how much they do achieve.'

Source: CHI Clinical Governance Review, 2001

Organisational culture

When we talk about 'organisational culture', we mean the values and beliefs espoused by an organisation. Culture has become known as 'the way we do things around here'. These 'ways of doing things' are not necessarily written down or explicit rules. They manifest themselves through the attitudes, behaviours and expectations of the people who work there.

For example, it is unlikely that there is a written policy about whether staff are permitted to question decisions made by managers in the organisation. But in most organisations, employees will know whether this is acceptable or whether it will be frowned upon. This is part of the culture of the organisation, and will affect the behaviour of staff. If questions from employees are dealt with in an open, co-operative manner, staff are more likely to ask for clarification again in future. However, if a query is met with a defensive reply, this is likely to discourage people from asking questions.

Everyone in an organisation influences its culture. Leaders and managers have a particular role to play. By shaping the culture in a positive way and setting the tone, they enable staff and teams to make their own contribution to improving

Joint clinical and managerial team work

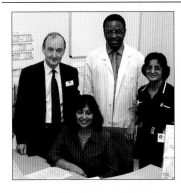

Photo: Clive Oakley, West Middlesex University Hospital trust

I was leading a pioneering scheme to improve cancer patients' care, creating a new breast and neurological clinic at the hospital. The project was one of 51 run by hospitals throughout the country, as a part of the cancer services collaborative that incorporated nine cancer networks.

The idea behind the scheme was to make the treatment of cancer patients much more efficient and friendly. If you look at it from their point of view they are handled by lots of different teams: GPs, outpatients booking staff, medical secretaries, X-ray staff and the waiting list office.

We found that a substantial group of cancer patients made a similar journey and therefore grouped together those with breast disease and neurological disorders. Previously they would have had to visit many different departments but we made it so the outpatient staff, the medical staff and the specialist nurses were all based in the same area.

By grouping together all the departments, we have stopped individuals working in the different areas blaming each other for mistakes or delays. For example, we had situations where the outpatient staff used to say that the medical secretaries had a patient's records when they couldn't find them.

As a leader I found that it was very important to get everyone in the team to respect each other's needs and create a shared sense of responsibility. Working as a single team also cuts down on administration, is much quicker and produces a much more patient-friendly system.

In the beginning it was hard to get staff to have confidence in the new way of working. To combat this we got people from different departments to sit down together and map the patient journey. What they found was that although the care the patient received from each department was good, the procedure as a whole was a shambles.

From a leadership perspective I had to encourage staff to trust each other to fulfil their part of the process. Now there is a huge sense of satisfaction in the team rather than each department working separately.

Hugh Rogers, consultant neurologist and clinical director of surgery,
West Middlesex University Hospital trust

services and promoting health. Culture is very much determined by how people interact with one another.

Tribalism

The NHS is often called a 'tribal' organisation. This refers to the many diverse professions comprising the healthcare system, and the fact that they all tend to have a slightly different view about care processes and clinical needs. In the past, the strong identities of single professional groups have reinforced the differences between colleagues and in some cases have been detrimental to patient care.

In addition, there have been tensions in the past between managers and clinicians in the health service. Much of this stems from the establishment of health service general management in 1983, when many non-clinicians took on wide-ranging responsibilities for healthcare organisations, leaving clinicians feeling threatened and powerless.

Huge efforts have been made to reverse these negative trends, which have proved divisive and which have hindered co-operation and progress in many parts of the health system. In recent years, there has been an increased emphasis on the need for partnership working across disciplines, across professions and across organisations. This is based on the premise that all professions and agencies have a part to play in shaping and delivering effective healthcare.

Importantly, this approach acknowledges the interdependence of different professional groups and stresses that more can be achieved by working together for the good of the patient rather than working to protect personal or professional interests. Excellent work has been done in many places to involve clinicians in decision-making and to support managers to better understand clinical issues.

When mistakes happen

The NHS has been criticised in the past for fostering a 'blame culture'. This is an environment in which mistakes are followed by the questions 'whose fault was it?' and identifying 'who was wrong?' Clearly, this sort of reaction to an error, mistake or accident will inevitably create a culture of fear among staff. People are likely to be afraid of making mistakes, and worried about reprisal if they do make an error. The long-term implication is that employees are likely to try

Leading through adversity

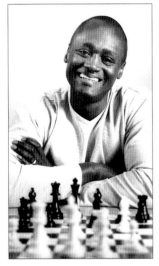

Photo: Sarah Hannant

During my career, I have been faced with a £3 million deficit when I started my job as director of finance at Central Middlesex and from there became involved in its merger with Northwick Park.

The NHS needs more than a skilled workforce and more than managers who are able to set targets, manage progress and review objectives. Leadership, for me, is this missing bit – people at all levels who can make us feel a sense of purpose in what we're trying to achieve, enthusiasm for a particular direction or solution.

My view of what leadership in the NHS entails has changed as my career has progressed. Early on, I think I confused a manager with a leader. You can have great leaders who are bad managers. Leaders don't have to be responsible for managing any staff.

Although I was involved in dealing with the £3 million deficit at Central Middlesex Hospital, I couldn't begin to take the lion's share of the credit for turning things around. I think that there were a few important factors. Firstly, the Central Middlesex community was pretty much united by a feeling of fighting for survival. Next they trusted the chief executive and bought into his values. Thirdly, I got some help from some contracted-in 'rottweilers', who could allow me to emphasise the picture, while they drew blood in their search for that extra few thousand.

This enabled me to fulfil my leadership role by emphasising the vision, emphasising why success was important, clarifying the nature of the problem and being passionate about the need for success and the future that would come with a new shiny building called the ACAD.

I didn't really need to motivate my staff at Middlesex, as when it comes to something as serious as that all finance staff are pretty motivated anyway. But I guess what I tried to be was more confident about success than I really was. Also, as this was a top priority, there was no problem with motivation. Being clear about the process from beginning to end was important.

In very difficult times, such as at Middlesex, I maintain my own self confidence by trying to refer back to the purpose of the NHS and constantly asking myself why I'm doing what I'm doing.

Trying to look at things from a reasonable point of view helps – it's not always good to rely on the way things have always been done. It helps to bounce things off other people to check if you're being reasonable. If all else fails a beer or two after work convinces people that they've got all the answers right.

I'd like to be as energetic and enthusiastic as I am on my good days all the time. Then I could say that my leadership style is confident, but reasonable, practical and yes, enthusiastic. I try to keep things light hearted but with high standards because I want people to enjoy being at work, then we all get better results. I try to remember what someone once told me, that leading is an art not a science.

Don Richards, director of finance and information technology,
North West London Hospitals trust

to conceal errors, which may in itself be a risk to patients. The whole culture of the organisation is likely to become one where people are 'watching their backs' and primarily protecting their own interests.

Becoming a learning organisation

'Becoming a learning organisation is more of a journey than a destination.'

Mike Pedler [3]

A series of high profile inquiries into serious incidents over recent years has highlighted just how widespread this culture of fear and reprisal has spread in the NHS. The inquiry into children's cardiac surgery at Bristol and the Alder Hey case concerning organ retention are just two examples. The introduction of clinical governance is an attempt to avoid these sorts of incidents in the future. However, for clinical governance to be successful, the NHS needs to develop a much more open, transparent and blame-free culture. It is vital that reporting errors and learning from mistakes is encouraged, in order to continually improve services, and for all staff to work together constructively to ensure the highest possible standards of care.

One of the key aims of clinical governance is to create a 'learning organisation', namely an organisation which is constantly ready for change, evolution and transformation. Learning organisations are those that support staff to bring about change and to continuously improve what they do. They provide a safe environment in which staff can take considered and measured risks, innovate and try out creative ideas with the aim of enhancing quality. Mistakes and errors are viewed primarily as a chance for further learning. This leads to a continuous cycle of learning and improvement. The resultant 'learning loop' is not just a single loop, where people learn whether something works or not. The exploration of why an approach did or didn't work creates 'double-looped learning' – firstly about the outcome and secondly about the reason for the outcome. This allows lessons about good practice to be embedded into everyday work.

Within a learning organisation, everybody has some responsibility and accountability.

Individual responsibilities in a learning organisation

- Engage in organisational dialogue to continually examine the worth of the organisation's purpose.
- Bring the best available knowledge to bear on organisational issues.
- Function as a co-participant in the creation, maintenance and transformation of organisational realities.
- Willingly share what each knows with colleagues and create forums and systems to accomplish this.
- Actively learn from experience every day to develop as a responsible, participating member of the organisation.
- Share in the responsibility for the governance of the organisation.

Source: N Dixon, 1998[4]

The role of the board in a learning organisation

At the highest level of a learning organisation, research suggests that the board should be giving thought and consideration to how it spends its time, dividing its attention between the following activities:

Accountability	**Policy**
- Patients, users and clients - Public - Staff - NHS Executive - For ensuring direction	- Creating vision, values and culture - Stating purpose - Maintaining external environment
Monitoring	**Strategic thinking**
- Overseeing management - Maintaining budgetary control - Maintaining other results, ie activity, quality, patient satisfaction **From: Garratt, 1997[5]**	- Planning to achieve the vision - Reviewing and deploying resources - Identifying current capabilities - Creating a synergy, service plans, HR plans, capital plans, etc

This is highlighted by Nancy Dixon in her consideration of the responsibilities of individuals in learning organisations.[4]

Within the context of the NHS, reflective practice is an example of a system that supports the principles of a learning organisation. This provides time to review the effects of clinical practice, consider whether anything could be done differently and assess how everyday clinical practice can enable everyone involved to learn in an ongoing manner.

Significant event audit

This is a way of looking at events – good and bad – to see how care can be improved. Patient or team experience can be looked at in a systematic and supportive way, promoting a shift away from hierarchical to more democratic team processes.

This structured method has been mainly tested in primary care and allows trust to be built so that the team can focus on 'what is wrong' rather than 'who is wrong'. Details of the technique can be found at http://latis.ac.uk/sigevent/

A learning organisation positively embraces the need for continuous change. Research undertaken into highly performing teams showed that principled leadership was a critical factor in determining the success of teams. The relationship between leadership and culture are shown in the box below.

Leadership and continuous improvement

- To achieve an elevated goal or vision, change must occur.
- For change to occur, a decision must be made.
- For a decision to be made, a choice must be made.
- To make a choice, a risk must be taken.
- To encourage risk-taking, a supportive climate must exist.
- A supportive climate is demonstrated by day-to-day leadership behaviour – by setting an example.

From: Larson and Lafasto, 1989[6]

REFERENCES

1 O'Rourke A. *Accountability* Wisdom Centre, Institute of General Practice & Primary Care, Sheffield University. 2000. http://www.wisdomnet.co.uk

2 DoH. *A First Class Service: quality in the new NHS*. Stationery Office. 1999.

3 Pedler M. A Guide to the learning organization. *Industrial and Commercial Training* 27 (4) 21-25. 1995.

4 Dixon N. The responsibilities of members in an organisation that is learning. *The Learning Organization* 5 (4) 61-167. 1998.

5 Garrratt B. *The fish rots from the head – the crisis in our boardrooms: developing the crucial skills of the company director*. Harper Collins. 1997.

6 Larson C, LaFasto F. Teamwork – *What must go right, what can go wrong*. Sage, London. 1989.

Notes

"If you think you can or you think you can't, you're right."

Henry Ford

Developing yourself as a leader

Introduction

Having provided some context and background about leadership in the previous section, this chapter focuses on your own development as a leader. It aims to help you identify your current skills and strengths, and to become aware of the gaps in your knowledge or skill-set. Practical strategies are then suggested for developing your effectiveness as a leader.

Just as for practitioners, ongoing personal and professional development is the key to achieving excellence as a leader and manager. There are a range of development programmes, qualifications and courses which can be useful to support leadership development (see page 150 for useful contacts). In addition, you may find support for your development in the workplace, in the form of discussions with your manager, performance appraisal systems and access to courses and development. 150

See CD-ROM for HSJ articles 'Getting into the swing' and 'Governing the guv'nor'

Effective personal development

The importance of building the skills and awareness to develop your own effectiveness as a leader cannot be underestimated. Leaders who know and practise the art of 'self-development' are well equipped to excel in their work and to provide inspiring role models for others.

There are other important reasons why it is essential to concentrate time and effort on self-development:

- Training courses and qualifications can only go so far in supporting your development. Your effectiveness at work relies on learning by doing, from successes and mistakes. Your own experiences at work are a source of powerful learning – but it requires thought and commitment to maximise this.

- Career paths are no longer as pre-determined and predictable as in the past. Employability, based on a set of transferable and relevant skills, is becoming the key influence in people's career progression, and movement between organisation types is much more frequent than in the past. Self-directed development can help to ensure that you remain 'ahead of the game'.

- Few organisations are in a position to respond to all staff development needs, due to the wide range of skills and talents among staff, and the variety of different 'career directions' they are likely to take. While many organisations can provide a 'springboard' for your development, the extent of your progress is largely up to you.

- Personal development as a leader is much more than keeping up-to-date with relevant issues. The development of personal competence is just as vital, and this is, by definition, an on-going, proactive activity that you are best placed to initiate.

Above all, becoming self-directed in your personal and professional development helps you to improve your work performance, enhance your career prospects, increase your capacity to learn and gives you increased confidence to deal with the continual change of today's working environment.

- Development should be continuous in the sense that the individual should always be actively seeking improved performance.
- Development should be owned and managed by the individual.
- Personal and professional development is an individual matter and the effective learner knows best what they need to learn.
- Regular investment of time in learning should be seen as an essential part of professional life, not as an optional extra.
- The emphasis should be on learning from an extremely wide range of activities.
- Work should be seen as a key learning experience and opportunity.
- There should be an emphasis on outcomes – answering the questions 'what did you learn from this experience?' and 'how can you apply this learning?'
- Learning objectives should be clear and wherever possible, should serve organisational as well as individual goals.

Adapted from *Policy and Guidelines on CPD,* Chartered Institute of Personnel and Development, 1997

Sources of learning and development

'I am always willing to learn, but I do not like being taught.'

Winston Churchill

Learning and development can be derived from many different sources, and it is worth considering a wide range of options when planning your approach. The first thing to decide is whether your development requirements can be met within the workplace or whether you need external stimulus.

Work-based development activities integral to your work might include:

- Running a training event for colleagues.
- Implementing new systems for doing things.
- Project work, to undertake a specific piece of time-limited work.
- Writing reports.
- Making presentations.
- Coaching or mentoring a colleague or member of staff. (See section in Chapter four page 70.) →70
- Obtaining a mentor. (See section on mentoring page 52.) →52

- Inter-departmental 'shadowing' to find out about others' roles.
- Secondments.
- Attending meetings or forums you are not usually involved in.
- Membership of committees or groups which inform decision-making.
- Visits to other organisations.

See CD-ROM for an HSJ article about shadowing: 'The book of revelations'

Outside of work, possibilities include:
- Public duties, eg – school governor, non-executive director.
- Voluntary work.
- Membership of clubs/societies.
- Writing or lecturing.
- Pursuing hobbies/interests.
- Reading.
- Attendance at seminars/conferences.
- Undertaking qualifications.

Try to think as imaginatively as you can about ways in which you can develop your talents and build your confidence. Of course, the more you enjoy the activity you choose, the more you are likely to learn from it.

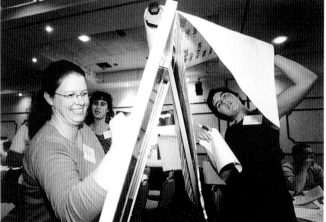

Learning and development can be derived from many different sources. The HSJ Future Leader's Challenge gives younger staff a taste of leadership at senior level.

However, sometimes it is necessary to move outside your natural 'comfort zone' of activities you enjoy, in order to stretch yourself and push your personal boundaries.

Learning styles

Reading through the lists of possible development activities, it is likely that some appeal to you far more than others. This is partly due to the fact that everyone has a preferred learning style, or approach to learning. Some people like to learn by being thrown in at the deep end and getting on with the job. Others find they learn more effectively

Four learning styles		
Learning style	**Learn most from activities which:**	**Learn least from activities which:**
Activist	Provide new experiences Contain excitement and drama Are varied Give you some of the limelight Allow you freedom to explore Throw you in at the deep end Involve other people	Involve a passive role Require you to 'stand back' Involve lots of data Are solitary Are theoretical Require practice Involve precise instructions
Reflector	Allow thought and reflection Involve observation Provide time to prepare Involve indepth fact-finding Allow review after the event Are structured and planned Are not time-pressured	Give you the limelight Require immediate action Are unplanned or impulsive Provide partial information Provide precise instructions Are rushed or pressured
Theorist	Are part of a concept or theory Allow a methodical approach Involve logic and analysis Are intellectually challenging Are structured Involve reading and researching Involve complexity Which are relevant to the job	Have no apparent context Emphasise feelings or emotions Involve ambiguity/uncertainty Scratch the surface Appear methodologically flawed Seem superficial Involve less academic people Are not of immediate use
Pragmatist	Provide practical techniques Allow you to practise Provide an example to follow Give immediate chance to try out Appear of practical application	Appear theoretical Lack guidance or demonstration Are time-consuming Do not seem relevant to real-life
		Source: Honey and Mumford, 2000[1]

if they can think through an issue or situation before taking action, or perhaps they like to see the practical application of any learning before they value it.

Being aware of your preferred learning style can help you to identify activities that will be of most benefit to your own personal development. It can also help you to consider other people's learning styles, which can be useful when working with colleagues and staff members in addressing their own development needs.

Honey and Mumford have developed a questionnaire to help you identify your own learning style, which also provides suggestions about how to make your learning more effective.[1] A summary of this is provided in the box opposite.

Personal development planning

When thinking about personal and professional development, it can sometimes be difficult to know where to start. A structured and systematic approach can help break down the whole process of personal development planning into manageable chunks.

There are five steps to creating a personal development plan:

1 Do a stock-take of your current skills, ability and knowledge.
2 Set objectives for what you want to achieve in terms of work, lifestyle and personal goals.
3 Identify the areas you need to develop in order to achieve your goals.
4 Decide on the steps necessary to address your development needs. You can do this by drafting your development plan.
5 Review on an on-going basis.

Activity 1

Identify your personal learning style. Use this information and the framework described above to draw up your own personal development plan. Think about ways in which you can best implement it.

Your personal development plan will be based on addressing the identified 'gaps'. Your plan does not need to be documented, but doing so

See CD-ROM for further guidance on producing a personal development plan, and a suggested format

can help to structure your thoughts and also enables you to measure your progress – which can be quite encouraging.

Your leadership style

There are many technical management skills which are the nuts and bolts of a manager's job. These skills need to be developed over time, often taught and learnt, and most certainly practised. In addition, a vital component in the leader's toolkit is the 'can of oil', which can often make the most tricky and difficult tasks just a little easier to handle. In the case of leadership, the can of oil equates to a high level of self-awareness and an understanding of how to achieve a continual and fruitful process of self-development.

There are a range of questionnaires available, which can be completed to identify your style and approach to management and leadership. Some of the better known ones include the Myers Briggs Type Indicator™ (MBTI), the Leadership Practices Inventory (Kouzes and Posner 1996), and the Multifactor Leadership Questionnaire (MLQ, Bass & Avolio 1995). These are often used as part of leadership development programmes, as the feedback usually needs to be given by a person trained in the use of the questionnaire.

See CD-ROM for a straightforward questionnaire that can be used to identify a key element of your leadership style

Whilst formal tools and techniques such as questionnaires can help provide insight into your own leadership style, they cannot paint a full picture. Some of these approaches are based simply on your own assessment of your style. While this is valid and important, the way you see yourself often differs from the way in which others perceive you. To become more aware of yourself and your behaviour at work, it is extremely valuable to gain the views of those around you.

360 degree feedback

360 degree appraisal is a relatively new organisational and personal development tool and is becoming increasingly popular. There are a range of instruments available and a number of specialist consultants who can

develop systems for your organisation. However, once you understand the principles, there is nothing to stop you developing a local approach to suit your situation, perhaps with the help of expertise in your organisation.

The term '360 degree appraisal' generally refers to a formal process of feedback on an individual's performance, using a structured questionnaire to gain the views of a range of people including the individual concerned, their line manager, peers, direct reports and internal and external customers. The questions are normally linked to a set of competencies or job-related factors with the individual playing a key role in deciding who takes part in the appraisal.

Feedback from the questionnaire is analysed and reported back to the person concerned. Feedback may be attributed or anonymous, depending on the system used. Individuals are usually given a structured opportunity to respond, and are encouraged to share the feedback with others.

360 degree appraisal can be a powerful tool when used as part of a comprehensive approach to organisational and personal

development. However, it can have a negative effect on individuals and organisations if implemented in the wrong way. See the tips on page 51 on introducing an effective 360 degree appraisal system. → 51

If you want to know more, a good place to start is your own human resources department, or the person who is the personal and organisational development lead in your organisation.

A couple of organisations have done some very well-regarded work on 360 degree appraisal. For example, South Tees Acute Hospitals NHS trust has done some notable work with clinicians. Gloucester Health Authority has been awarded beacon status for their work on appraisals including 360 degree feedback.

The tips on page 51 apply to introducing 360 degree appraisal to a whole organisation. While it is ideal to use a 'tailored', competence-based instrument for this, there may be a range of reasons why this is not possible or realistic. Don't let this put you off the idea of 360 degree feedback. As an individual or team leader, you can encourage your team members to be receptive to feedback from others, and you can lead the way in this through your own approach. See the section on constructive feedback' for more details on this. 67

See CD-ROM for HSJ article 'Turned to good account'

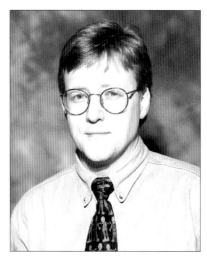

Approaching a 360 degree exercise for the first time is a daunting prospect. Asking those you manage, those who manage you, your colleagues and those who receive your services for feedback on how they see you can be quite a challenge.

However, in this era of clinical governance such openness, honesty and courage to grow is not only desirable but necessary. Like many of my colleagues in public health I have had to rapidly develop new areas of competence over the last couple of years as I have engaged with an ever-widening agenda. This has involved dealing with new issues and forming new partnerships. There has been little time for formal training, guided development or reflection.

The 360 degree exercise therefore gave me the chance to check out how I was being perceived and gain feedback on those areas I intuitively felt that I was performing well in. It also gave me the chance to check out others' perceptions of areas I wasn't so comfortable with.

For me, the most important part of using 360 degree feedback is the chance to illustrate to my staff and colleagues my own willingness to model the way and embrace the culture of on-going learning and improvement.

Andrew Rogers, health promotion manager, West Pennine Health Authority

Introducing a 360 degree appraisal process: some tips

- Think about the whole process before you start. What is your organisation's culture and what are you trying to achieve through this process? Remember that the system for devising and sustaining personal development plans is as important as the process for carrying out the initial appraisal and giving feedback to individuals.

- The process is most likely to succeed if commitment comes from the top. If the chief executive and senior management team are willing to go through the process themselves, the system will have more integrity.

- Remember that the cost in time, money and administrative effort can be considerable. Don't think about introducing a system until you are sure your organisation can handle this. Make sure you use a reputable instrument that is relevant to your organisation's needs. Generic or 'off the shelf' systems may not be right for you and you may need to budget for a tailored approach. Any new system should be piloted, preferably with senior management, before being rolled out. There needs to be extensive training on interpreting results, giving and receiving feedback, and developing personal development plans.

- 360 degree appraisal systems work best when based on competency frameworks linked to organisational objectives and as part of wider performance management and personal development strategies. Systems based on salary or bonus schemes, or linked to redundancy or promotion issues, tend to work less well, because there is more pressure on colleagues to respond in a certain way.

- Not all organisational cultures can support the introduction of 360 degree appraisal. The system tends to work best in open, learning-based cultures where there is already an emphasis on communication and an atmosphere of trust and support. In organisations characterised by competition or a 'blame' culture for example, the introduction of 360 degree appraisal may exacerbate rather than change the prevailing way of doing business. If you think your organisational culture may not support the introduction of such a system, it may be better to work up to its development rather than going for a 'big bang' approach.

- 360 degree appraisal systems cannot shore up existing failing systems of appraisal. Used well, they are a complement but not a replacement for wider processes of appraisal and performance management. No system, however good, is a substitute for addressing underlying issues of management and leadership in your organisation.

If you are the subject of a 360 degree appraisal, or receive any other form of feedback from others, you may find the following tips useful.

- Don't overreact to criticism. Most people find receiving feedback a daunting prospect. Remember the process known as SARA: shock, anger, rejection, acceptance. Don't make it SARAR (revenge). Try to put it in context.

- Look for discrepancies between how you have scored yourself and how others rate you. Many people rate themselves more highly than others do. You can expect to get the toughest ratings from direct reports, as they see more of your behaviour. Don't overemphasise the importance of your manager's ratings – they're just one part of the total picture.

- Ask yourself what you see in these patterns. For example, if your peers rate you more highly than direct reports, are you spending more time and skill influencing them? Look for overall patterns. What are your greatest strengths and biggest development needs?

- Don't dismiss the positives as 'things that anyone can do'. What you find easy, others could find hard.

- Think about what you are going to do about the feedback and what action planning you will do to feed into your personal development plan.

- How will you give people feedback on what they've told you? The brave thing to do is copy the whole report and discuss it with them. If you can't face that, a summary is better than nothing. The most important thing is to ask for clarification and specific examples.

- Finally, remember feedback is not an instruction to change. You have the choice about what you do next.

Mentoring

The origins of mentoring are in Greek mythology. Before Odysseus left for his epic journey, he entrusted the care and upbringing of his son to his learned and trusted friend, Mentor. Trust and learning are still very much associated with the term 'mentoring' and this approach to development has become increasingly popular in recent years. A mentor is often an integral part of a formal development programme, but a mentoring arrangement can be set up completely independently.

People choose to find a mentor for a variety of reasons. Having a mentor is essentially about forming a relationship with someone who can help you to develop, who is not directly involved in your day-to-day work. Ways in which they can help your development might include: sharing their experiences, helping you to reflect on your work, offering insights, challenging your viewpoint, providing access to contacts and networks, helping you to think things through, discussing issues, suggesting development opportunities – the list could go on.

What is mentoring?

Whilst the possible ways of using a mentor are extremely diverse, there are some key skills and attributes to look for in a mentor:

- Someone whose personal qualities you admire.

Mentoring is about	Mentoring is not about
Getting advice	Becoming dependent
Furthering your development	Managerial supervision
Building trust	Power and hierarchy
Learning from others' experience	Winning or losing
Building your confidence	Sticking to comfort zones
A non-judgemental approach	Feeling exposed or compromised
Developing an on-going relationship	Control
Hearing a different perspective	A 'free ticket' to anything
Exploring options	Being told or instructed
Airing opinions	Lecturing
Gaining knowledge	Hero-worship
Learning about influence	A one-off meeting
Stretching comfort zones	What the mentor needs
Extending your networks	
Being challenged	
What the 'mentee' needs	

- Experienced and knowledgeable.
- Someone you can trust.
- A willingness to commit long-term.
- A commitment to developing others.
- Effective feedback skills.
- Accessibility and approachability.
- Excellent interpersonal skills.
- Preparedness to challenge.
- Good communicator.
- Organisational understanding.
- Clarity and focus.
- Sensitivity to changing needs and circumstances.

Identifying an appropriate person to be your mentor is worth careful thought. You may want to ask other people for suggestions or recommendations. Some organisations have lists of people willing to be mentors (ask the HR department). If you are unable to identify anyone yourself, and your organisation is unable to help, there are companies who specialise in matching you with a mentor who can help your personal development. Your HR department should be able to supply you with information about these companies.

Most people are flattered to be asked to be someone's mentor. But both people involved need to enter into the agreement willingly. It is a good idea to make an initial approach in principle, and suggest to a potential mentor that the two of you meet up to discuss each other's

Choosing a mentor

At the beginning, I had to pluck up the courage to ask her to mentor me. But I think having a good mentor is one of the most important things you can do for your own development.

The important thing is to choose carefully. You have to connect as human beings and, though you set clear boundaries, you can't put up barriers – you have to be prepared to disclose something of yourself.

Often I'll talk about something that's come up and she will recount a similar experience of hers and describe how she handled it. Sometimes she'll challenge me over something I've done or said, but it's always in a positive way. She makes suggestions and like everybody, I tend to procrastinate, but she'll always pick me up on it next time and asks me what I've done about it.

Nurse and counsellor

expectations before making a commitment. It is important that you both feel enthusiastic and clear about the relationship. It is also essential to agree ground rules about things such as:

- Confidentiality.
- Frequency and timing.
- What happens if it doesn't work.
- Expectations of each other.
- What your needs are as a 'mentee'.

See CD-ROM for an HSJ article on mentoring: 'Head to head'

Effective networking depends on two-way relationships.

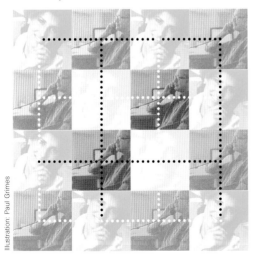

Illustration: Paul Grimes

Building your networks

'In organisations, real power and energy is generated through relationships. The patterns of relationships and the capacities to form them are more important than tasks, functions, roles and politics.'

Margaret Wheatly

As a leader, you are part of a wide network of people who all play a role in shaping ideas, developing services, building organisations and leading people; in short, a network of leaders at all levels, including many people with similar professional interests as you. Whilst you are part of this network in theory, proactive steps are needed to link yourself into the network in practice. This is known as 'networking'.

The purposes of networking are varied, but can include:
- Getting to know 'who's who?' in your field of interest.
- Raising your own profile in your field of interest – getting your name and face known by others.
- Learning from what is happening elsewhere.
- Sharing good ideas and approaches with others.

- Understanding how the 'jigsaw' fits together in your area of interest.
- Identifying who the key people and leaders are in your field.
- Exploring possible career options.
- Making contact with people who may be able to help you in the future.
- Offering help to others for the future.
- Keeping up-to-date, maintaining your personal and professional development.

It is important to remember that networking depends on lots of two-way relationships; to successfully develop your network, you need to be prepared to give and take – to share as well as to ask for support or information. Do not underestimate what you have to offer to others. People are often interested to hear how things are done in other organisations, and what may seem commonplace to you might be a new idea for other people.

Ways of developing your networks:

- Attending conferences or seminars, where other attendees are involved in similar work to you, but perhaps work in other parts of the country.

- Joining professional bodies. These organisations have wide membership and organise events and activities to help members meet each other and benefit from each other's experience. Professional bodies also often support professional development activities.

- Taking the opportunity to attend meetings concerning your areas of interest.

- Identifying specific people locally who could provide you with advice, help or information. (Remember that most people are pleased to offer their expertise and skills to help others.)

- Subscribing to professional journals and identifying names of people who are active in your area of interest, for future reference.

- Contacting writers of journal articles to find out more. Most people who write in professional journals are keen to spread the message about what they are doing.

- Consider contributing to a professional journal yourself, eg – by writing a letter or article describing good practice where you work.

- Letting people know that you are happy to be contacted to share any information and experience you have.

Developing your networks

 Leadership in the public sector is at a watershed. In producing the NHS plan, the government has come up with probably the most far-reaching programme of reform for healthcare services in the world. It is aiming to provide the sort of flexible and responsive service that has eluded most post war governments. To do this effectively will require magnificently good leadership.

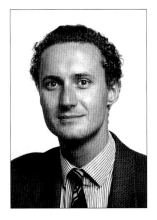

When I was on the NHS management training scheme, I used to think that there was a top secret course that trained you to become a leader. I now understand that it's about your personal capacity to lead. I believe that leadership is about the clarity of your vision and mission combined with unswervingly strong values. You then need to be able to communicate all that in a way that people engage with. Networking and mentorship is key to this. It set me off on a highly beneficial journey that has helped both my leadership and personal development.

I started to network at an early age. Through the MTS, I was able to meet high quality managers and leaders. Early in my career, I presented to a group of Australian healthcare executives and as a result of that managed to wangle an invitation to work in Australia for six months. This showed me how things can be done differently and made me look at the NHS through fresh eyes when I returned.

The NHS is target driven but during my middle management years I was fortunate enough to work for fantastic people who have given me the support, freedom and confidence to meet these targets. I also made an effort to meet people with different thought processes to myself which enabled me to look at issues from a range of different perspectives.

I still network now I am at senior management level. I tend to do this by having regular quarterly dinners with three people whom I respect and trust. I also receive formal coaching. I have found the challenges and support this offers tremendously helpful, particularly during my transition to chief executive status. I am also fortunate enough to have twice yearly mentor meetings with Nigel Crisp when we can exchange thoughts. I also make sure that I get 360 degree feedback on both my performance and my personal style.

My advice to anyone seeking to develop themselves as a leader would be to find people you trust and admire. Don't be afraid or bashful. Most people will be flattered if you approach them and ask for their help, advice and support. It is very important that when so much pressure is on us, that we still find the time and strength to develop our networks and our relationships.

Mark Britnell, chief executive, University Hospital Birmingham NHS trust

Developing your emotional intelligence

'Anyone can get angry – that is easy. But to get angry with the right person, to the right degree, at the right time, for the right purpose, and in the right way – that is not easy.'

Aristotle

Effective leaders are able to foster pride and purpose in their teams, to motivate them as well as improve their performance. Concentrating on the people side of the leadership equation by developing your emotional intelligence will help you to do this.

Emotional intelligence is the ability to sense and understand both your own and other's emotions and to apply that understanding to influencing and achieving your desired outcomes. It stems from studies undertaken in the US by Mayer and Salovey in the early 1990s that aimed to develop a way of scientifically measuring the difference between people's ability in the area of emotions.[2] They found that some people were better than others at things like identifying their own feelings, identifying the feelings of others and solving problems involving emotional issues.

The term 'emotional intelligence' became common currency in 1996 when Daniel Goleman – taking his lead from Mayer and Salovey – published a book under this title.[3] According to Goleman, emotional intelligence can be broken down into a number of components:

- Self-awareness – recognising your own strengths and weaknesses and knowing how to compensate for them.
- Managing your emotions – this is about self control, thinking before acting and keeping your emotions in check.
- The ability to motivate yourself – your optimism and personal drive to achieve a goal.
- Empathy – being able to read the emotions of others and to understand their motivation.
- Building and managing relationships – how you handle the emotion of others.

Work carried out by the Hay Group, one of the world's largest human resource consultants, showed that emotional intelligence is twice as important as cognitive abilities in predicting outstanding employee performance and accounts for more than 85 per cent of star performance in top leaders. Strong interpersonal skills are crucial for leadership success.[4]

Developing your emotional intelligence underpins and reinforces much of your personal leadership development. It is not something you can expect to become expert in overnight. Research suggests the best way to improve your emotional intelligence is to undertake a long term development programme with specific and achievable people management targets and objectives. This programme should encompass coaching,

feedback, encouragement, peer support and modelling in addition to on the job practice.

You can test your emotional intelligence levels at the Hay Group website. http://ei.haygroup.com/resources/library.html

Learning leadership from others

'If you want to see change, be the change you want to see.'

Ghandi

This chapter has provided a flavour of what leadership is and has outlined ways in which practitioners and managers at all levels in an organisation can develop themselves as leaders, and in so doing, make a noticeable difference to the way things are done.

The ideas, tools and techniques described in this section are all designed to help you gain more understanding of what leadership means for you in your work, and how you can develop as an effective leader. At the heart of all the approaches described is an acceptance that you are responsible for your

Emotional intelligence is about understanding and sensing both your own emotions and the emotions of others. You can use this understanding to achieve desired outcomes.

Photo: EMAP Healthcare Open Learning/Richard Smith

own personal development and that becoming a good leader is a process of on-going learning.

One final source of learning and development worthy of a mention is perhaps the most accessible and convenient of all. Learning by watching others can be a powerful way of observing how different people lead. The 'modelling' technique, whereby you model your approach on that of someone else, can be an effective way of extending your own repertoire of leadership skills and behaviours.

'Modelling' does not mean simply copying somebody else – this would probably not feel very comfortable, and is likely to appear unnatural or inconsistent. Rather, modelling involves identifying elements of the way others do things which you respect and admire, and considering how you can introduce these aspects of behaviour or approach into your own work.

Everyone has their own leadership approach, and 'modelling' is another way in which you can identify and nurture your personal leadership style. Remember, too, that as a leader, you offer a role model to others. The old adage is that actions speak louder than words – and being an effective leader is much more about showing leadership through demonstrating it rather than talking about what leadership is. This is also known as 'walking the talk'.

Activity 3

1. Write down the names of one or two people whose leadership style you really admire.

2. Try to observe these people in action – listen carefully to what they say, how they say it, what they do and how they treat others. Keep a note of the things you observe which sum up the reasons you appreciate their style.

3. How can you incorporate some of their approach into your own work?

REFERENCES

1 Honey P, Mumford A. *The learning styles questionnaire: 80-item version* [and] *The learning styles helper's guide.* Peter Honey Publishing. 2000.

2 Salovey P, Mayer JD. Emotional intelligence. *Imagination, Cognition, and Personality,* 9, 185-211. 1990.

3 Goleman D. *Emotional Intelligence.* Bloomsbury. 1996.

4 'What makes great leaders – Rethinking the route to effective leadership.' *Fortune magazine,* Hay Group; Executive survey of leadership effectiveness. 1999.

"The leader does not take on the mantle of magician him or herself but persuades followers that they – and only they – can resolve the problems they face."

Strengthening leadership in the public sector [1]

Developing others

Introduction

Managers of teams are often engaged in 'staff development' activities, which can range from discussing an individual's development needs, undertaking appraisals, supporting staff in training and development opportunities to coaching and mentoring staff, to name but a few. Within organisations, there is usually some sort of training and development department, which also provides resources and expertise in personal and professional development, and often in organisational development, too.

This chapter intends to provide practical approaches to supporting the development of others, and helping people to become more self-sufficient in managing their personal and professional development. There are also sections on how to facilitate effective appraisal processes and how to encourage a climate of constructive feedback.

Supporting the development of others

Part of the essence of leadership is about enabling others to perform to their best, to fulfil their potential, and to become leaders in their own right. An effective leader recognises that each individual's development is ultimately their own responsibility, and that the ability to develop oneself as a leader is one of the keys to becoming more effective. All the principles and approaches to development discussed in Chapter three 'Developing yourself as a leader' (see page 41) also apply to developing other people in your team. **41**

Successful leaders also acknowledge that they have a key role to play in supporting individuals and teams in their personal and professional development, and in their development of leadership skills. They encourage people to take responsibility for self-development, and act as an agent and catalyst along the way.

The classic managerial model for developing people in organisations links an individual's development objectives to those of their department and then into the overall strategic objectives of the organisation. (See box page **66**)

There is a neat logic to this approach, which attempts to align the needs of staff members, the needs of their teams and service and the requirements of the whole organisation. This model is the basis of most staff development or appraisal systems, and provides a solid building block to underpin a leader's role in supporting the development of others. However, whilst developing people in their current role and organisation is important, a good leader also considers a person's wider development needs – in the context of the person's future hopes and aspirations – which may extend beyond the current organisation.

Effective appraisal

Appraisal is sometimes referred to as a 'performance review' or a 'personal development review', but the process is similar in most organisations. A formal appraisal discussion is usually carried out annually, although informal appraisal ideally takes place on a continuous basis throughout the year.

Features of an effective appraisal discussion

- *No surprises*
  Feedback during the year from the manager to individuals should include praise for good work and when performance has been below the required standard, a discussion to identify problems and find ways of addressing these. If this is happening effectively throughout the year, there should not be any big surprises for either person at the appraisal discussion.

- *Clear objectives*
  One of the outcomes of the appraisal should be some clear, agreed objectives for the future.

- *Manager acts as 'guide' rather than 'judge'*
  An effective appraisal takes into account the appraisee's own assessment of their performance as well as that of other colleagues and their manager. The manager's role is to guide and advise the member of staff about how they can fulfil their own potential and ambitions.

- *Focus on the future*
  Performance over the past year will provide the context for the discussion but should not dominate; good and poor performance should have been appropriately handled at the time rather than stored up for discussion in the appraisal. A focus on the future brings a positive, developmental flavour to the discussion.

- *Focus on behaviours, not personalities*
  Discussion of performance should relate to what a person needs to do in order to meet their objectives, rather than on the qualities they ought to have. This is discussed further in the section on constructive feedback – see page 67

- *Two-way dialogue*
  The appraisal is a discussion, not an interview. The process is designed to ensure that the appraisee takes an active role in the appraisal discussion and the objective-setting process.

- *Training is provided*
  The skills required to lead an effective appraisal discussion need to be developed through training and practice. Training will also benefit the appraisee, so that they are fully aware of how the process works, and how they can best plan for and participate in the appraisal discussion.

See CD-ROM for tips on writing objectives

Pitfalls to avoid in appraisals

- *Lack of planning*
  A good appraisal requires forethought and planning by both appraisee and appraiser. Consider what you wish to discuss in advance of the meeting.

- *Apologising or making excuses for the appraisal process*
  Instead, stress how important it is for every member of staff to have some dedicated time to discuss themselves and their job.

- *Using the appraisal for managing poor performance or for salary negotiations*
  Underperformance should be dealt with as a separate process, at the time it occurs.
  Salary negotiations should not be discussed during the appraisal, as this can detract from an open and honest dialogue about the appraisee's needs.

- *Talking more than the appraisee*
  It is important that the discussion balances contributions from you both, and that the appraisee has the chance to fully state their point of view.

- *Interruptions*
  Ensure that the discussion will not be interrupted by telephones, messages etc.

- *Dealing with negative issues first*
  Focusing on the 'positives' first helps to create a developmental climate.

- *Forgetting development needs*
  Make sure that there is time to discuss development needs as well as future objectives.

- *Feeling obliged to agree a list of training courses for the appraisee*
  Remember that development comes in many forms other than training courses, many of which are more beneficial. Encourage the appraisee to consider how best they can meet their development needs.

- *Avoiding important issues*
  If there are issues you are not confident to discuss, do not avoid them. Seek help and advice in advance to help you decide how you can effectively discuss these with the appraisee.

- *Forgetting the paperwork*
  It is important that the outcomes of the appraisal are recorded in writing and agreed between the appraiser and appraisee. This ensures that you and the appraisee can build an ongoing record of his or her progress, and use the notes of the appraisal to support his or her work.

Developing people in organisations: the organisation strategy approach

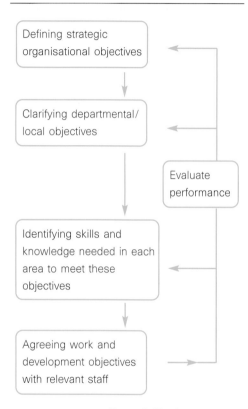

From: R Harrison, 1992[2]

The formal appraisal discussion gives a member of staff and their line manager the chance to step back from day-to-day work, take stock of how that person's job is going, and plan how the member of staff can be supported to

develop the job and themselves further. The main elements of an appraisal discussion are summarised in the box below.

Elements of an appraisal discussion

- What did you set out to do during the past year?
- To what extent did you achieve this?
- What factors had an impact on what you have achieved?
- What are you going to be doing over the next year?
- How will we know when you have done it?
- What support will you need to help you achieve this?
- What development will you require to help you achieve your more long-term goals?

It is important to differentiate an appraisal from the process of 'managing performance'. There is a separate process for managing poor performance, and an appraisal discussion is not the appropriate arena for initially raising these issues. You should ensure that you have undergone training in your organisation's procedures for dealing with poor performance.

The outcome of an appraisal discussion should help both the appraisee and the appraiser. The member of staff being appraised should know what is expected of them, what they need to do to achieve their objectives, and how they aim to develop their role and skills. The appraiser should know what the organisation can expect from the member of staff, what resources will be required to support the person to achieve their objectives, and how this will fit into overall organisational aims.

Activity 1

Find out about the appraisal system in your organisation. Gather any documentation, guidance and forms used as part of the process and if necessary, speak to your HR department to clarify how the system works. Ideally, you should attend a training workshop to help you to develop your appraisal skills; these are often provided in-house by the training department.

See the CD-ROM for a sample appraisal form, which you can use or adapt if your organisation does not have a standard one and for an HSJ article on consultant appraisal – 'Turned to good account'

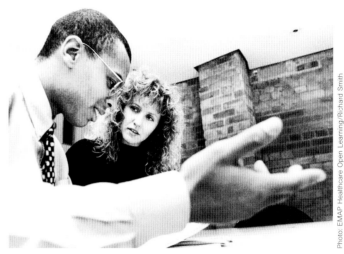

Effective leaders foster a culture in which giving and receiving feedback is an accepted and valued part of everyday life at work.

Constructive feedback

While it is important to make time for the formal appraisal of your team members, effective leaders foster a culture in which giving and receiving feedback is an accepted and valued part of everyday life at work. Feedback is one of the most valuable tools in a leader's toolkit, and underpins many of the core elements of effective people management. Constructive feedback helps create a culture where learning and continuous development are a priority, where positive work is highly valued and where mistakes are viewed as an opportunity for learning and improvement. It also fosters two-way, open communications and can encourage and motivate staff to continually strive for excellence.

An environment where constructive feedback is the norm cannot suddenly be created on a Monday morning. If people have not been used to giving constructive feedback to others or receiving much in the way of feedback themselves, then it will take time to help people to feel comfortable with the approach. However, the benefits of fostering such a culture are worth the effort. You may find that you need to start 'modelling the way' in offering feedback and asking for feedback from others, to demonstrate its benefits and encourage others.

Most people enjoy receiving praise and positive feedback, as long as it is sincere, but perhaps find that it does not happen very often. This is rarely because they are failing to do good work, but because colleagues are not in the habit of praising each other. If people make the effort to do so, they usually find giving positive feedback to another person a rewarding experience, as it tends to be well-received.

As a leader, one of the simplest ways of motivating staff and helping them to feel valued is by telling them about the things they are doing well. Staff who frequently receive positive messages about their work are more likely to feel that their contribution to the organisation matters. They are also less likely to feel demoralised if there is negative feedback every now and again, as it is in the context of lots of positive comments.

Negative feedback can be difficult both to offer and to receive in a constructive fashion. However, as stated in Chapter three (see page 43), self-awareness is one of the mainstays of developing oneself as a leader, and receiving constructive feedback is an excellent way of enhancing your insight into how others perceive you. Besides, before you start to offer feedback to others, it is highly advisable to ensure that you know how it feels to be on the receiving end. 43

Tips for giving constructive feedback

Do	Don't
• Ask the person if you can offer them some feedback.	• Comment on things that the person cannot change (eg, their accent).
• Base your comments on observations and facts.	• Leave feedback until a formal appraisal meeting.
• Provide specific examples about the exact time or behaviour you mean.	• Judge the whole person on the basis of their behaviour.
• Focus on behaviour, not personality – what people do, not who they are.	• Make a statement and then soften or retract it.
• Provide feedback as soon after the event as possible.	• Beat around the bush.
• Maintain an adult-to-adult, respectful manner.	• Give someone negative feedback in front of others.
• Give feedback frequently and informally.	• Avoid difficult issues or leave an issue unresolved.
• Be non-judgemental.	• Insist that the recipient must change.
• Balance positive and negative.	• Bombard the person with lots of feedback at once.
• Ensure feedback is a two-way dialogue.	• Offer feedback unless it is to help the other person.
• Leave the recipient free to decide whether or not to accept/act on the feedback.	• Suggest how things might be put right unless the person has accepted the feedback.
• Offer feedback in amounts the recipient can learn from.	• Adopt an 'I know best' attitude.
• Encourage the person to clarify what you mean.	• Tell people off.
• Consider how you would feel to receive the feedback you are giving.	• Make vague statements or sweeping generalisations.
• Listen carefully to the person's response.	• Criticise the person – only their behaviour.
• Be prepared for 'unexpected' reactions.	• Labour the point.
• Maintain eye contact.	• Give up if faced with initial resistance.
• Maintain a calm manner.	
• Clearly state your view.	
• Encourage the person to accept praise.	
• Encourage the person to gather further feedback.	
• Remember that tone of voice is as important as the message itself.	
• Let the recipient know how the behaviours made others feel.	

→

Activity 3

Think of a situation at work in which you feel you could improve your skills or performance (perhaps doing a presentation or chairing a certain meeting). Choose a colleague whom you trust and ask them to observe you in that setting, and to give you some feedback about how you performed.

Stress to them that you want to hear both complimentary and critical comments, so that they do not feel awkward. Try to learn from the feedback itself, but also consider how you felt when receiving it.

Are there any lessons you can learn from this about how to – and how not to – give feedback to others?

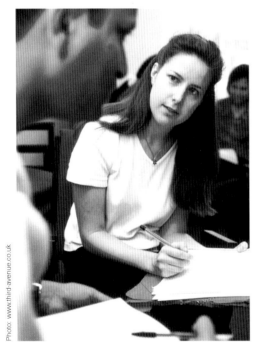

Photo: www.third-avenue.co.uk

Coaching is a process of using work opportunities to help people learn, supporting them in improving their present performance.

Coaching

'Coaching remains the secret weapon of many outstanding organisations. There is only so much that a business can productively do by way of down-sizing, restructuring, focusing on the core business and the like. Ultimately, it comes down to people – building winning teams.'

John O'Burdett [3]

Coaching is a well-known activity in the world of sport, and is increasingly used in organisations, too. The principles of coaching great sports champions are transferable to the development of people in the workplace. The person being coached is hungry to excel, has belief in their own abilities and is prepared for hard work, but acknowledges that they cannot achieve their ambitions on their own. The coach has not necessarily achieved what their protégé dreams of achieving, but has the required insight, knowledge and motivational skills and focus to propel them rapidly forward.

What is coaching?

Coaching is a process of using work opportunities to help people to learn, supporting them in improving their present performance. The focus is not about teaching someone how to do something, but tends to be about further improving the performance of somebody who is already performing well.

There are many benefits to staff of a coaching relationship with either their manager or someone else with relevant experience and expertise:

- It links learning directly with the job.
- They can see the effects through their improved performance.
- It can improve motivation, interest and confidence.
- It recognises ability and develops skills.
- It is a process of continuous improvement.
- It offers regular and relevant feedback and review of performance.

Benefits for a manager and organisation can include:

- Improved performance.
- Better working relationships.
- More staff involvement.
- Improved communication.
- Shared aims and objectives.
- Enhanced team spirit.
- A sense of shared success.

Barriers to coaching

If coaching is new to you, you may have reservations or concerns. The coaching process certainly requires a willingness to open up the communication processes within your team, and to see your relationship with your team as one of continual development. Mutual trust between you and the receiver of coaching is fundamental to its success.

It is also important that you consider the impact of coaching on your own role. It will take time and commitment, and you may feel that you cannot afford this. Remind yourself that one of the most important things a leader does is to develop other leaders. Your team needs constant development in order to progress, and this requires time. The advantage of coaching is that the benefits are of immediate relevance to the job.

Another consideration is that with highly performing team members, your own role may change. For instance, it may become appropriate to pass over some of your own responsibilities to other members of the team. As they develop, they are likely to become keen to take on new areas of work. For you, this may mean giving up sole responsibility for work you particularly enjoy. However, if you are committed to developing others, you are likely to feel a sense of fulfilment in seeing the progress of your team. And remember, freeing yourself up from parts of your role gives you scope to develop new areas of work.

Potential obstacles to effective coaching might also exist in your organisation more generally. The 'culture' of your organisation might be one where managers are not familiar with the coaching approach, and are therefore somewhat suspicious, sceptical or resistant to the idea. (See page 32 for discussion of 'organisational culture'.) However, as a leader, you can certainly introduce coaching into your team and assess its impact. You may then choose to tell others

about it, and to demonstrate its value. 32

Equally, members of staff may need help to understand what is involved in receiving coaching, and to appreciate how it may benefit them. Your role will be to guide them in the process until they feel confident about it – in time, perhaps confident enough to coach others.

Agreeing an action plan for coaching

- What are the targets and aims?
- How will these be met?
- Who is responsible for which part of the process?
- What does the other person require from you?
- What do you expect of the person being coached?
- What immediate steps are needed by each of you?
- How will you know when progress is being made?
- What are the time scales?
- How frequently will you meet?
- What are dates and times of future coaching sessions?
- How will you communicate between coaching sessions if necessary?

Tips for introducing coaching

- Make time for a one-to-one discussion and ask the person about their view of their role and progress.
- Concentrate initially on existing strengths and how the person would like to build these further.
- Explain how coaching works and explore what this might mean for the individual concerned.
- Stress that the process will be shaped by both of you, and that their input and ideas will be central to this.
- Make sure the person has all the information they need to make their own decision about coaching.
- If necessary, provide time for the person to go away and think through what you have discussed before deciding to go any further. They may want to clarify their understanding of the process and purpose of coaching.
- Keep a clear distinction between coaching and other processes, such as appraisal or supervision. Whilst there may be overlaps, it is important that the coaching process complements rather than replaces other one-to-one discussions.

The coaching process

The first step in introducing coaching is to identify which of your team members would benefit, and which elements of the job would provide appropriate coaching opportunities. Activity 4 on page 74 provides a suggested starting point. **→74**

Once you have generated some initial ideas about the people and tasks that may be involved in coaching, the next step is to introduce the idea to others. It is essential to remember that coaching requires two-way commitment and interest, so keep an open mind at this stage. The people you have in mind may not respond as you expect, so it is important not to plan too far ahead before you have heard their point of view. Otherwise, they may feel that they are being expected to take part, rather than being offered an opportunity to do so.

Once you and a member of your team have agreed to start a coaching relationship, a focused approach will help to provide initial momentum, and to maintain on-going clarity. An action plan can help with this

There are also some practical things that you need to arrange. These include:

- An appropriate place to meet.
- Providing access for your member of staff to other departments and relevant information.
- Deciding how their new activities will fit into their current role.
- Making others aware as appropriate.

Once the coaching process is underway, you will need to allow your team member to explore their new opportunities in their own way. As a coach, you will need to keep a discreet eye on how they are responding to the challenges without being tempted to intervene prematurely. Of course, it may be that you need to step in if serious mistakes are likely, but try as far as you can to let your member of staff experiment and learn for themselves.

Frequent review meetings in the early stages can help you to assess the extent to which your direct input is needed. Remember that 'there is more than one way to skin a cat' and that your member of staff may do things differently from you, but may still achieve a good outcome. There is learning in this process for both of you.

Review meetings will be important to keep the process on track. These are most effective if they are informal and open, with the focus on learning and development. Your feedback skills and your ability to help your member of staff evaluate their own progress will be of

Activity 4

Give some thought to the following questions, and note down your responses.

Who in your team:

- Has clear further potential?
- Is motivated by achievement and progress?
- Seems ready for further challenge?

What elements of the team's work could provide a coaching opportunity? Eg –

- A specific project.
- Aspects of your job which you could delegate.
- Specific activities that could be further improved.
- Skills development which would widen the scope of somebody's job.

crucial importance in these meetings. Effective review meetings will highlight progress so far, identify problems and obstacles and celebrate success. They will also identify ways in which your member of staff can further practise and develop skills and tasks.

REFERENCES

1   Honey P, Mumford A. *The learning styles questionnaire: 80-item version* [and] *The learning styles helper's guide*. Peter Honey Publishing. 2000.

2   Salovey P, Mayer JD. Emotional intelligence. *Imagination, Cognition, and Personality*, 9, 185-211. 1990.

3   Goleman D. *Emotional Intelligence*. Bloomsbury, 1996.

4   'What makes great leaders – Rethinking the route to effective leadership.' *Fortune magazine, Hay Group*; executive survey of leadership effectiveness. 1999. http://ei.haygroup.com/downloads/pdf/Leadership%20White%20Paper.pdf

Notes

"A team is essentially a group with a common aim, in which the skills and abilities of the members are complementary."

John Adair

Building effective teams

Introduction

In most work environments, there are occasions when groups of people function as individuals and times when they work as a team. Even at those times when people can effectively work alone, it is usually important to consider the impact of individual actions on colleagues. In other words, most people belong to some sort of team, even if this is an 'extended' team rather than a close-knit one. Some people will belong to more than one team at a time, reflecting the different sets of people they work with in their role.

This chapter explores the nature of leadership within the context of a team and provides an opportunity for you to review your own approach to leading teams. This includes an overview of team development processes and an introduction to the roles individuals play within teams.

Leading teams

A group of individuals is not necessarily a team, but will benefit from working as a team in the following circumstances:

- When the task can be carried out by one person, but where there is not enough time for this – others are therefore needed to get the job done quickly, eg – sorting out medical records for a large number of patients.
- When the effort required in a task cannot be exerted by one person, eg – using certain patient hoists.
- When the task involves several distinct but simultaneous tasks, eg – emergency ambulance; all in the paramedic team may have the same skills, but none of them can drive the ambulance at the same time as treating the patient.
- When the task requires several different type of skills or knowledge, eg – a primary healthcare team, community mental health team.

Research has shown that the climate within a team can account for 30% of the team's performance. The climate of an organisation is the atmosphere or perceptions of a workplace. This includes the clarity with which people understand their roles and how they relate to the organisations' objectives, the performance

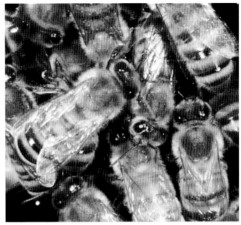

Effective teams will perform to their best and work with others to fulfill the organisation's purpose.

standards and expectations, the flexibility and lack of workplace constraints, the authority and responsibility people are given and how they are recognised and rewarded. The climate has a direct impact on performance. When climate changes are sustained over time, they can shift the organisation's culture. The leader of a team has a critical influence on this climate, and up to 70% of the organisational climate is influenced by the styles a leader adopts towards others in the team.[1]

A fundamental part of leadership is building a team of individuals who are motivated to perform to their best and who work effectively with others to fulfil the organisation's purpose. John Adair identified three key areas that need to be considered within a team. These areas are represented by three circles:[2]

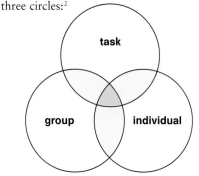

The leader has a key role to play in keeping the three elements carefully balanced. Over-emphasis on the task is likely to result in neglect of the needs of the group or individual team members. Likewise, too much focus on individuals within the team is likely to have a detrimental effect on the task and the overall group. If group needs dominate, there is a risk that individual needs and the achievement of the task may suffer.

Establishing ground rules for effective team work

Once you have built your team, it will function more efficiently if ground rules and team concepts are laid down and adhered to. These might include:

- Agreeing the goals of the team and the critical success factors it needs to achieve from the offset.
- Encouraging team members to think and talk in terms of 'we' rather than 'I' and to share a common language.
- Holding regular meetings and agree how long the meetings will last (not too long).
- Planning in a major team celebration at regular intervals.
- Using the team for real work: disseminating information, sharing good practice, solving problems and learning from each other.
- Planning thoroughly before acting.
- Speedy identification and resolution of group conflicts.
- Communicating effectively.
- Focussing team members on clients and customers, eg – patients, other teams within your organisation, partners outside your organisation.
- Using the team to identify issues that are causing problems, and act on your findings.
- Encouraging the team to regularly review its work and achievements.
- Leading by example.
- Helping balance to emerge between: team roles and functions; task and process; home and working life.

Teams: Three areas of need

Task

The need to accomplish something, eg – solve a problem, provide a service, make a decision. The need of the group is to try to accomplish this task and so long as this task remains undone, there will be a tension in the group and an urge to complete the task.

Group

The need to develop and maintain working relationships among the members so that the group task can be accomplished. Group needs refer primarily to people and their relationships with each other. It concerns how people relate to each other as they work on the group task.

Individual

Individuals bring needs with them into groups and teams. People work in groups not only to accomplish the task, but often because it fulfils a need in them as people, eg – social contact, sharing ideas, respect from others, a sense of fulfilment, being valued etc.

The individual is a key component of a group or team, and meeting individuals' needs will increase their motivation to contribute to the team. If such needs can be met along with and not at the expense of the task and group needs, then the team will tend to be more effective.

From: J Adair *Effective Teambuilding*, 1996

Of course it is unrealistic to expect all three elements to be equally balanced at all times. If a deadline is approaching, the task needs are likely to take priority. If new members join the team, group needs will require particular focus. If a key individual requires extra support, the needs of that individual will come first. But over time, an effective leader will be consciously attempting to balance all three sets of needs in order to optimise team performance.

Activity 1

Think of a team you lead or of which you are a member. Which of the three circles usually takes priority in your team? Why is this?

Which circles, if any, tend to be neglected in your team, and why? When does this happen?

How do you think you could make the balance of the three circles in your team more equal?

The importance of effective teams

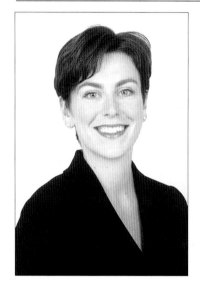

 A leader's job is to get results – but very few of these results will be achieved by the leader in isolation. Most results will be delivered by team members, so in order to do your job you need your team to perform well. An organisation such as a hospital relies on effective team work.

Teams are most appropriate for dealing with difficult and highly complex tasks, such as those involved in running a hospital. They provide the best way of working when consensual decisions are essential, when there is a high degree of choice and uncertainty and when a great deal of commitment and a broad range of competencies is needed from team members.

As a team leader, it is important to be focused and organised. Your attitude and values will influence team members considerably and illustrate your expectations of them. This is especially critical when, as in my case, the team consists entirely of other leaders. Your behaviour, standards, professionalism and enthusiasm will act as a guide both in terms of expected behaviour within your team and in leading their own teams.

You need to understand and value the individuals within your team and allow them to lead, too. It's important to give them the freedom to make decisions and to make changes within their areas of responsibility.

You should support your team both when things go right and when they go wrong. Most importantly, you need to allow your staff time to talk to you, so that you can listen, and understand their issues. By doing this you can help them realise their potential. If someone has made a mistake, then as the leader that is your mistake too and you must help them through it. If there is a performance problem you go through it privately and calmly. You treat team members with decency at all times, as you expect them to treat their staff in turn.

Teams go through different phases in their lifecycle and when a new member joins, inevitably the dynamics change. When I began in my current post I took over as team leader to an existing team. I could sense some trepidation about how I would lead them and compare to their last team leader, who had been very popular. Everyone was charming of course, but there was a degree of formality and reserve at putting forward views and suggestions. It wasn't long before people realised that they could express themselves freely to me and at this point team meetings became much more productive – and enjoyable.

Tara Donnelly, director of operations, Whittington Hospital, London

Team development

Newly formed teams have been shown to move through stages of development as the members become accustomed to working together, as shown in the box below. As a leader of a team, it is useful to be aware of these stages of development in order to understand some of the reasons why teams do not always work at their optimum level.

Some commentators have added the 'mourning' stage to the diagram. This acknowledges that a change in the team's membership can be a critical factor in how the team works together. If members join or leave the team, it may revert to an earlier stage of development, re-forming and progressing through the 'storming' and 'norming' phases again.

Stages of team development	
Forming Formation of team	Team members are finding their feet; identifying the task; establishing boundaries and rules; identifying what resources will be needed; getting to know each other; looking for guidance from the team leader; learning what behaviours are appropriate.
Storming Establishing relationships	A flaring-up of emotion and conflict; reaction against the demands or value of the task; conflict between sub-groups; challenges to the position of the leader; reaction against the demands placed on the individuals and team.
Norming 'Settling down'	Developing cohesiveness as a group; co-operating and exchanging ideas and opinions; laying down the standards, norms and expectations, encouraging mutual support.
Performing Real progress and results are achieved	Solutions begin to emerge; constructive work forges ahead; members take on positive functional roles; group energy is directed towards the completion of the task.
Mourning?	If the team composition alters, the team is likely to need to re-adjust and may revert to previous stages of development.

Based on a model by BW Tuckham, 1965[3]

An effective leader balances the need for these stages of team development with the need to achieve a 'performing' team as quickly as possible. Building in time devoted to team development can help the team to move to the 'performing' stage, and the team leader may decide to initiate some team development activities to facilitate this process.

Activity 2

Consider a team you lead or one in which you are a member. Identify occasions when it seemed that the team was at each of the stages identified in the box: **forming, storming, norming,** and **performing** on page 83

What behaviours could be observed in the team at each of these stages?

Has the team been through a mourning phase? How did this become evident in the way the team worked?

The point of team development is to enable a team to work more effectively together to achieve its aims. Approaches to team development take many forms, depending on the needs of the team and its stage of development.

Sometimes, teams that have been established for a while appear seem to have got 'stuck' and appear unable to make progress. This can be because the team has not been allowed to move through the 'storming' phase. Although this phase can be uncomfortable, it lays the foundations for subsequent team development, and a leader may instigate ways of encouraging the team into the 'storming' phase.

Other team-building work may focus on the 'norming' stage. This may involve identifying people's strengths, preferences and needs for support, sharing mutual expectations, comparing values and motivation and understanding the roles of each member of the team. This type of team-building is focused on establishing an agreed way of working together, based on the individuals in the team.

During the 'performing' stage of team development, an effective leader is likely to encourage the team to remain aware of its development needs in order to perform as well as possible. Team development work may focus on clarifying the task or purpose of the team, or reviewing the way the team is working and making any improvements to enhance its effectiveness.

When a team gets 'stuck'

 A new multi-disciplinary team offering an outreach substance misuse service had reached a critical stage in their development. All the team members had joined the 'pilot project' with high levels of motivation fifteen months earlier and they believed that they could develop exciting new ways of offering services, based on innovative approaches to care. They were all keen to evaluate the effectiveness of the pioneering approach they were taking. After just over a year, energy levels were flagging, and several members of the team were considering leaving. All team members felt let-down, disappointed and frustrated.

The pilot project was led by a clinical psychologist, and the other team members included a psychiatrist, community psychiatric nurses, occupational therapists and administrative staff. The clinical psychologist suggested an 'away day' to review the team's progress, and an external facilitator worked with the team to do this.

During the course of the away day, it transpired that this was the first time the team had sat down to discuss the way they were working together. Although they met regularly, there was always pressure to discuss the project and the evaluation work rather than to review the team processes. As a result, many misunderstandings had developed, and team members had grown suspicious and resentful of each other.

The away day focused on identifying people's feelings and views about the team from the beginning of the project to the present, in order to identify when problems had occurred. This led to honest and at times uncomfortable discussion about the way different team members had behaved on certain occasions, and it became clear that there was a fundamental lack of shared understanding about team members' roles within the team.

In particular, the leadership and management of the team was unclear to all members of the team. Most of them were under the impression that the clinical psychologist, as project lead, was their line manager and leader. During the discussions, it transpired that the clinical psychologist did not view herself as the team manager at all; simply as the clinical lead for the project. She told the team at the away day that she had no desire to manage the team. This basic misunderstanding helped to explain many of the problems the team had encountered. The work done during the day to clarify the roles of team members cleared the air, allowed for people's skills to be recognised, and laid the path for the team to move forward.

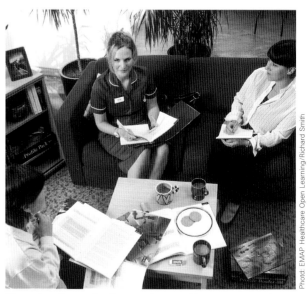

See the CD-ROM for a team-building exercise that can help to identify team values and develop awareness of group needs within a team.

Team roles

'A team is not a bunch of people with job titles, but a congregation of individuals, each of whom has a role which is understood by other members.'

M Belbin

Dr Meredith Belbin is a British researcher and writer who has spent many years exploring the way teams work. He has studied the way in which complex management problems are tackled in teams of varying composition. The managers' different personality traits, intellectual styles and behaviours were assessed during the exercises and different clusters of behaviour were identified as underlying the success of the teams.

From this work, nine clusters of behaviours emerged, which were classified into separate team roles, which are shown in the box on the opposite page.

Belbin describes a team role as 'a tendency to behave, contribute and interrelate with others in a particular way'.[4] The roles he has identified fall into three main categories:

- **Action-oriented roles** – shaper, implementer, and completer-finisher.
- **People-oriented roles** – co-ordinator, team-worker and resource investigator.
- **Cerebral roles** – plant, monitor-evaluator and specialist.

The point of team development is to enable a team to work effectively together to achieve its aims.

Belbin team types		
Belbin team-role type	**Contributions**	**Allowable weaknesses**
Plant	Creative, imaginative, unorthodox. Solves difficult problems.	Ignores incidentals. Too pre-occupied to communicate effectively.
Co-ordinator	Mature, confident, a good chairperson. Clarifies goals, promotes decision-making, delegates well.	Can often be seen as manipulative. Offloads personal work.
Monitor-evaluator	Sober, strategic and discerning. Sees all options. Judges accurately.	Lacks drive and ability to inspire others.
Implementer	Disciplined, reliable, conservative and efficient. Turns ideas into practical actions.	Somewhat inflexible. Slow to respond to new possibilities.
Completer-finisher	Painstaking, conscientious, anxious. Searches out errors and omissions. Delivers on time.	Inclined to worry unduly. Reluctant to delegate.
Resource investigator	Extrovert, enthusiastic, communicative. Explores opportunities. Develops contacts.	Over-optimistic. Loses interest once initial enthusiasm has passed.
Shaper	Challenging, dynamic, thrives on pressure. The drive and courage to overcome obstacles.	Prone to provocation. Offends people's feelings.
Teamworker	Co-operative, mild, perceptive and diplomatic. Listens, builds, averts friction.	Indecisive in crunch situations.
Specialist	Single-minded, self-starting, dedicated. Provides knowledge and skills in rare supply.	Contributes only on a narrow front. Dwells on technicalities.

Source: M Belbin

As a leader, it can be useful to use the Belbin team type framework with teams to help them analyse the membership of the team. This can be done using the Belbin test, a questionnaire that identifies the preferred roles of each member in a team.

It is important to remember that a team benefits from each of the Belbin roles, and that no individual role is more or less important than another. Indeed, Belbin's research suggests that a team lacking some of the roles is likely to perform less well than a team where the members can fulfil all the roles effectively.

It is worth remembering that a team role is a tendency to behave in a certain way, but that it does not preclude other behaviours. Most people have a preference for how they would usually behave in a team, and this is highlighted by the Belbin questionnaire. One of the benefits of the Belbin framework is that is can help a team identify where its strengths and weaknesses lie, and how any weaknesses can be addressed.

The strengths of team members can then be used to positive effect, while team behaviours which do not come naturally to team members can be borne in mind, and appropriate steps taken to make up for this.

For instance, a team may discover that none of its team members is a strong 'completer-finisher'. This may help to explain why the team gets through a lot of work, but finds itself having to go back to previous jobs and tasks to refine work or correct mistakes which were originally overlooked. The team could use the Belbin framework to decide how it can compensate for the fact that nobody in the team is a natural when it comes to attention to detail.

You can find a link to www.belbin.co.uk on the CD-ROM

Activity 3

Consider the descriptions of the Belbin team roles shown in the box on page 87. For each member of your team, identify which team role best describes the way they tend to behave in the team. How many of the team roles do you think are present in your team? Remember that one person may demonstrate more than one natural team role. 87

REFERENCES

1 Performance and Innovation Unit. *Strengthening leadership in the public sector.* 2000. http://www.cabinet-office.gov.uk/innovation

2 Adair J. *Effective teambuilding.* Gower; London, 1986.

3 Tuckman B. Developmental sequence in small groups. *Psychological Bulletin*, 63, 1965: 384-389

4 Belbin RM. *Management teams - Why they succeed or fail.* Butterworth Heinemann, 1981.

Notes

Communicating and influencing

Introduction

Many of the problems that occur in an organisation are the direct result of people failing to communicate. Bad communication can cause many problems. It leads to confusion and can cause a good plan to fail.

This chapter considers the role and skills of communication in leadership, and provides a framework for using these to develop your awareness and effectiveness in influencing others.

Leading communication

Communication is important at all levels and for all people in an organisation. Leaders arguably have a particular role to play as 'sense-makers' and 'sense-givers'. Sense-making involves converting complexity into something understandable, giving focus to ambiguity and translating uncertainty into clarity. Sense-giving involves communicating a direction, a purpose or a vision which connects the 'now' with the future. All these types of communication are needed in an organisation, and are most likely to come from the leaders.

A large part of any leadership role is achieved through influencing and persuading other people, and by 'making things happen' through others, rather than necessarily doing things yourself. Communication strategies are central to effective influencing.

Consider these questions:

- How do people make sense of their departments and organisations?
- How do individuals at work communicate and understand each other? What language do they use? Do they talk in terms of 'I' or 'we'?
- Why do individuals at work sometimes fail to understand each other?
- What role do leaders play in making sense of the work environment?
- Is the leadership role to help others make their own, but shared, sense of the work environment?
- How can organisations develop meanings, visions, a sense of common purpose, understood and shared by all staff?

These are just some of the questions which illustrate why communication is so central to leading an organisation or team. As a manager and leader, you rely on communication to fulfil your role. The keys to effective communication are **what** you communicate and **how** you communicate it. Other important factors include the style in which you communicate, how often you communicate and consideration of whether the communication is a two-way process, or whether you want to convey information directly to its audience.

What leaders communicate

The type and amount of communication in which leaders engage are determined by their own style, their skills and by the culture of the organisation. According to Adair, there are three levels of perceived need for communication:[1]

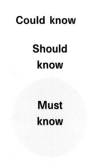

Could know

Should know

Must know

The more open and communicative the culture within an organisation, and the higher the priority given to keeping people involved, the more likely an organisation is to fulfil all three levels of communication need. In a more restricted, closed culture where communication tends to be top-down, the focus is more likely to be limited to the 'must know' and 'should know'.

Activity 1

Consider how you decide what to communicate to your team or colleagues. Would you say that you respond to their 'must-know' needs only, or to their 'should/could know' needs too? What are the advantages of your approach? What are the drawbacks?

If your team or colleagues are deciding what to communicate to you, at which level of communication would you wish them to operate? Would you prefer them to communicate about things they think you 'could know', 'should know' or just about the things you 'must know'?

Is there a match between what you expect from others and what you provide to them in terms of communication?

Congratulate yourself if there is a good fit, but often there are considerable gaps. Being precise about these helps you to address communication problems. A good way of identifying the gaps and problems so that they can be addressed is to carry out a communications audit. This can take a number of forms, but it is usually helpful to:

- Identify your audiences, both inside and outside your workplace and think about how you would like to communicate with them.

- Identify what methods are currently used to communicate with your audiences and what methods you would like to use.
- Identify how your organisation or team encourages feedback from its audiences.
- Identify what your audiences see as effective communication tools, eg – people might not like the use of e-mail because it takes up a lot of time replying to messages and because there is no personal contact involved.
- Consider what is cost-effective, eg – there is no point in spending a lot of money on an expensive newsletter if no one will make the time to read it.
- Think about what you could do better within budgetary and time limitations.
- Pull all the information you have gathered into an implementation plan that includes clear time scales and allows feedback. Start your improved communication campaign by distributing the plan.

How leaders communicate

Everything you say and most things you do are a form of communication, direct or indirect, conscious or sub-conscious. Yet only 7% of communication is verbal. Whenever you set out to communicate a message, the

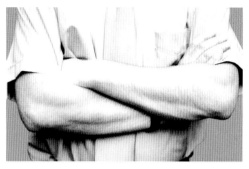
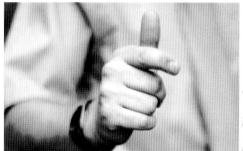

Photos: Rhiannon Frost

Everything you say and most things you do, including your body language, is a form of communication.

receiver will perceive both content and context. Whether or not you realise it, messages and meaning are constantly present in all your behaviour, and this can be as powerful, if not more so, than the words you actually say.

Given the significance of communication to your effectiveness as a leader, it is worth putting effort into ensuring that effective communication systems are in place.

However, it is not easy to remain in constant contact with people, particularly if you work in different physical locations or if the teams you lead are widely dispersed. Although technological developments have contributed to enabling more remote, electronic communications, these provide an alternative mode of communication rather than replacing any of the more conventional forms. Every form of communication has both benefits and drawbacks.

The proof of whether communication is successful lies in its impact, not in its intent.

Activity 2

Consider what the recipient's reaction is likely to be in these three examples:

- A carefully worded e-mail to tell a member of staff that they are being made redundant.
- Reading out a well-written report in a meeting.
- Leaving a clear written note for somebody to explain why they were unsuccessful in an interview.

What would be a more appropriate means of communicating each message, and why?

Leadership communication – lessons from the communication industries

It can be useful to analyse how the communication industries convey their messages. You will often find ideas you can use yourself.

Advertising – The advertising industry finds a clear message and repeats it often. It uses multiple media to send out the same message and it finds ways to measure its results.

Television – The television industry schedules communication slots and aims for regularity. It uses narrative and story telling.

Film - The film industry finds inventive ways to capture undivided attention. It segments target audiences, eg – by age.

Source: Getting the attention you need – Davenport and Beck (*Harvard Business Review*, Sept-Oct 2000)

A well-meaning approach to communication is in itself not successful; the impact it has on the recipient is the most critical issue.

Choosing an appropriate means of communication is the key element that determines the impact of the message.

Examples of a poor match between the mode of communication and the message illustrate this point. In the examples given in Activity 2, the 'intent' of the communicator is likely to have been well-meaning, but the 'impact' is unlikely to have been positive. Despite the quality and clarity of the message, it is the mode of communication in these examples which leads to ineffective communication. **96**

Of course, communication is a two-way process, often involving many people, and the importance of receiving a message is central to how effective you are as a communicator. The box below provides some of the keys to effective listening.

Communication styles

The style of communication adopted by a leader often reflects their overall leadership style and the way they interact with their staff and colleagues. The box on page 100 shows some of the features of 'open' and 'closed' approaches to communications. There are benefits and drawbacks to both approaches, and most fall somewhere in between. You can begin to develop your awareness of this by observing the style of communication used by leaders in your organisation. It may be useful for you to consider whether you think these styles are suitable in the circumstances, and why certain styles are adopted. **98**

Effective listening

- Be willing to listen: this requires an open mind and a willingness to be influenced by what you hear.

- Hear the message: includes listening to the words, picking up non-verbal signals and putting effort into understanding the message, 'listening between the lines'.

- Interpret the meaning: run through the message with the person presenting it, to ensure you have interpreted it in the way it was meant.

- Evaluate carefully: assess the worth or value of what you have heard.

- Respond appropriately: to ensure that the communication is two-way. Responses may include comments, questions, non-verbal responses.

- Anticipate the reaction: consider how your response may be received and be prepared for this.

Open communication	Closed communication
• Promotes co-operation, working relationships and information flow. • Staff who have contributed to the organisation's plans are likely to understand the aims and work towards them. • More likely to instil a sense of self-worth, mutual trust and confidence. • Enables others to speak out without fear of reprisal. • Mutual working towards common goals – better motivation. • Problem-solving, openness and honesty, empathy, egalitarian. • Influenced by management style, history and previous experience. • Takes time and effort.	• Information is power – withholding information can increase control. • Can lead to territorial behaviour, possessive attitudes. • Can be mechanism to ensure conformity. • Can be used to conceal a hidden agenda. • Emphasises status and differences. • Characterised by lack of discussion, lack of compromise – one way messages. • Saves time in the short term.

Activity 3

Think about how you communicate with your staff and your colleagues. Write down two or three examples of when your communication style featured characteristics of:

a) open communication

b) closed communication

What are the reasons for the different styles on different occasions?

Influencing others

A large part of any leadership role is achieved through influencing and persuading other people, and by 'making things happen' through others, rather than necessarily doing things yourself. You are likely to need to influence in all directions:

Upwards – to manage the expectations and to influence the view of your immediate manager and others more senior to yourself.

Dealing with the media

If you are a leader at a junior or middle level of your organisation, it is unlikely you will be called upon to deal with the media. But as you progress up the career ladder, you may find contact with the media becomes more frequent. These tips will help you.

- If it is part of your role to speak to the media, make sure you have professional media training. This will make you feel more confident, less likely to panic and give you an appreciation of what the journalist is looking for.

- Make sure you prepare properly before you take part in an interview. Research what the journalist wants to know before you meet them. Put yourself in their shoes and think about the issue from their perspective. This will help you to identify and anticipate any difficult questions that are likely to be asked.

- Tell the truth. In moments of stress it can be tempting to try to deflect the questioner, shift the blame or even to lie but the best policy is always honesty.

- Think about what you want to say and rehearse it. Try to come up with some pithy sound bites as what you say, particularly on television, is likely to be edited. Use anecdotes if appropriate. Ask someone else to listen to you to make sure you are making sense.

- If you have to buy time to think, prepare a phrase in advance. Be aware that the phrase 'well, I'm glad you asked me that' has become a cliché.

- Resist the urge to become hostile if the journalist is taking a difficult line of questioning. Remember that the journalist is only doing their job and the media is your only line of access to current and potential patients.

- If you are appearing on television, think about what you are wearing. To be taken seriously you need to be dressed seriously so play down the bright colours and complicated hairstyles.

- Take a proactive approach and build up relationships with local journalists. This way you will hopefully be given the opportunity to put across your viewpoint first. However, don't have favourites. If you give an interview to one paper, you must be prepared to give one to every paper.

Downwards – to persuade those who report to you or who are less experienced or senior, to join you in pursuing an idea.

Across – to gain support from other parts of the organisation, and from peers and colleagues at a similar level to yourself but with different professional backgrounds.

Inter-agency – to build allegiances and effective working relationships with colleagues working in other agencies in the health community.

You are likely to have a preferred style of influencing, and it is useful to become aware of this when considering how you can further develop your influencing skills.

See the CD-ROM for an influencing style audit questionnaire, which will help you to think about how you influence other people, and how you can improve your skills

Influencing people at work

The following section deals with key factors that are important to bear in mind when considering how to influence others at work.

Status
Attitudes towards seniority and hierarchical position vary considerably among managers, and these are often influenced by the culture of the organisation. Generally speaking, it is useful to take status into account in deciding how to influence another person, and modifying your approach accordingly. As a leader, try not to allow status to influence the content of your approach; if you have a point to make, then it is valid to do so regardless of the other person's status. It is likely that how you deliver the message will be the key to how it is received. Remember that bad news can be effectively and skilfully delivered, and good news can sometimes be poorly handled.

If you are in a more senior position than the other person in a discussion, it can be helpful to consider how that person views your status, and whether this may affect the way they behave with you.

Communication for clarity

 Where communication is concerned, it is important that there is no dislocation between leaders and other staff. A leader doesn't necessarily have to completely understand what others are doing but they must have a sense of what is going on, and an appreciation of any problems they may have. I think a breakdown occurs when leaders become aloof and separated from their staff, this is when they stop being a good leader.

A leader should be accessible and take time out to explain what they're doing. A good leader should inspire questions from their staff. You often find bad leaders push their staff away because they don't want to be troubled with trivia but the questions asked of a good leader aren't usually of this nature because the leader has given people the confidence and ability to do their job well.

I have quite an easy-going style of communication with my staff but I have very high expectations of them. The ethos I use is that I appoint good staff and I expect them to do the job well.

At CHI we have a very open relationship and my team know they can come to me at any time with any problems or ideas they have. I see our relationship as very much a two-way thing. I strongly believe in praise where it is due – people are often too busy to tell someone they've done a good job. But when people could be doing something better, I address that too. I also expect my team to tell me if they thought I was doing something the wrong way and I will listen to their suggestions.

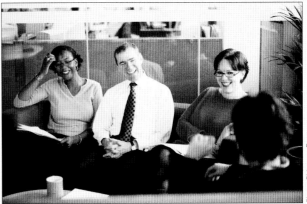

Photo: Rhiannon Frost

When I speak to staff at different levels in the organisation I'm trying to achieve different things. When I speak to the senior managers at board meetings I'm looking to influence strategies and plans in terms of the big picture. When I speak to my own staff I am less strategic and more concrete in what I want them to achieve. I use a similar approach with both groups, it's just that the nature of what we need to discuss is different.

Communication between different bodies is absolutely fundamental. I regularly speak to others in a similar position to me in other health related organisations, such as the Modernisation Agency. People within my organisation also regularly speak with their opposite numbers and we meet up around every six months. It is part of our duty to make sense of all the different opinions and information for everyone working in the NHS.

Matt Tee, communications director, Commission for Health Improvement

Ask yourself:

* What do I know about this person's attitude towards status and how can I adapt my approach accordingly?

Organisational power

In most organisations, there are people who are known to have more influence than others. This is not always related to seniority or position. For example, certain people may have unique expertise meaning their views are respected, or they may have a network of contacts from a previous job, which can help your own organisation.

Try to familiarise yourself with who the key influencers are in your area of work and, where possible, find out what this influence is based on. It can be useful to gain the support of such people when trying to influence others. However, you will probably want to think carefully about how you do this, and how it might be perceived by others.

Ask yourself:

* Is the person I am trying to influence connected with organisational power, and if so, how might this affect their view?
* Are there people in the organisation whose

support would help to strengthen my case?

Personal relationships

It is very useful to think about your interaction with another person in the context of your previous encounters with them. If you have worked with the person before, you will have views and feelings about them, which may affect the way you try to influence them. For example, if they have made life difficult for you in the past, you may fear this will happen again, and find yourself being cautious in your discussions with them.

Similarly, you may benefit from considering your likely relationship with them in the future. It can be tricky to balance the need to 'keep people on board' and maintain long term constructive relationships whilst trying to influence people in the short term. You may need to weigh up how important an immediate issue is and how likely it is to affect your future working with this person.

Ask yourself:

* How will my previous knowledge of this person affect my approach to them?
* How might my approach impact on my future working relationships with this person?

Successfully influencing others

 As a PCG chair, the people I need to influence depend on the particular issue in hand, but may include the entire local population, the borough council, the county council, the regional office, the health authority, local trusts, all members of local primary healthcare teams, social services, voluntary organisations, Uncle Tom Cobley and all.

An example where all these players have been involved is our consultation process to move to PCT. This has not been helped by a neighbouring PCG (another group to be influenced) lining up their borough councillors and voluntary organisations to oppose our progress. Another factor that has added to the difficulty has been the health authority's apparent failure to deliver the relevant information to the appropriate people. Social services have also been 'playing games' at a senior level which adds to the frustration. It is fascinating how everyone who stabs you in the back does it in the name of partnership and improved inter-agency working.

An example of a successful influencing strategy was in getting seven out of the 10 practices in the PCG to switch to personal medical services. This was achieved by working with an outside 'expert' who was perceived by the practices as both knowledgeable and neutral.

Having sown the seeds and disseminated detailed information to all the GPs, a meeting was called with several experts on a panel to answer all their questions. This not only gave them the detailed information that they needed, but allowed them to voice their anxieties – and they certainly did.

Follow-up meetings involving all the practices gave the project an impetus and as it moved forward through these it became less likely that people would opt out.

It helped that individuals saw clear benefits for them, but as with so many initiatives the detailed financial information required was only available at the 13th hour. Fortunately, by this stage the group's motivation to move forward was so strong that even the financial hiccups were overcome.

GP and chair of PCG

Timing

It may seem an obvious point to make, but timing can be crucial when trying to influence someone, and this can be worth some prior consideration. Approaching a person with an idea or proposal when they are in the middle of dealing with an urgent issue or when they appear pre-occupied is unlikely to yield positive results, and may jeopardise your chances of influencing them.

It is worth trying to plan some dedicated time to discuss key issues with the people you wish to influence, and think through the approach that you are going to take. In the usual course of events at work, it is possible that occasions arise when it seems appropriate to begin the process of influencing others in an informal and unplanned manner, and it is important to look out for such opportunities.

Successful influencing

The process of influencing others is often based on building ongoing effective working relationships with people, through which you earn respect, credibility and a good reputation, rather than through a one-off discussion. This reinforces how important it is

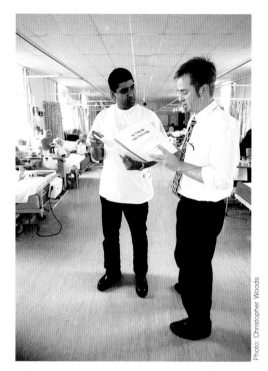

Photo: Christopher Woods

The process of influencing others is often based on building ongoing effective working relationships with people.

to be as aware as possible of your leadership behaviour and of the impact it has on others.

It is often said that the best proof of effectively influencing others is when somebody you have spoken to about your idea brings it to you as a proposal. This may happen months later, but you can be sure that you played a part in shaping thinking about the issue. Although you may not get the credit, as a leader you can take pleasure in seeing others feel positive about an idea, and be supportive of this. If others see that you appreciate good ideas, they are more likely to make positive suggestions in future.

Classic approaches to negotiation and influence stress the principle of aiming for a 'win-win' result (see figure below). Steven Covey in his book *The seven habits of highly effective people* describes win/win as a process of co-operation that seeks to give equal benefit and opportunity to all parties involved in the change process, enabling them to feel committed to the action plan.[2]

This is helpful as a reminder that getting everything your own way in a discussion is not necessarily a good outcome, if it leaves the other person feeling that they have conceded on every point. You may feel that you have 'won' but the other person is likely to feel that they have 'lost' (you lose I win). The repercussions of this could be wide-ranging, but may involve the other person feeling resentful, or being reluctant to discuss issues with you in the future.

The reverse of this is that you may concede all your points of a discussion to the other person, and end up feeling as if they have 'won' everything and you haven't won anything (you win, I lose).

In some circumstances, the discussion may become complicated, and the outcome may be that neither of you leaves feeling that you have achieved anything positive (lose-lose). In these circumstances, it is important to review and understand why this has happened, and what you could do to avoid this happening again. This might involve altering your approach to the other person, reviewing your expectations of the discussion, planning ahead before the discussion or adopting a different influencing strategy.

		You	
		Win	**Lose**
Me	**Win**	You win, I win	You lose, I win
	Lose	I lose, you win	I lose, you lose

The ultimate success in influencing others, whether in discussion or negotiation, is to reach a point where both you and they feel that the outcome is positive and fair (win-win), given the circumstances and issues involved. It may be that each of you has had to make some concessions or have had to agree to a compromise of some sort. Whilst this may feel less than perfect, the key to gaining agreement is the sense of balance and fairness that the compromise and concessions have been made on both sides rather than just one side.

Finding a win-win

When a north London trust was undergoing a reconfiguration process, a member of staff resisted the change because she was not a confident driver and was worried about travelling by car to the new site. After discussing this with her, her team leader suggested that the trust could pay for the member of staff to have refresher driving lessons to boost her confidence. This was arranged and the member of staff was happy with the arrangement. She coped well with the change in site and also felt motivated by the fact that her team leader had listened to her concerns and taken them seriously.

Activity 4

Think back to a recent discussion when you were trying to influence someone. Imagine the possible outcomes of that discussion in relation to the matrix in the box on page 105, eg – what would an 'I lose, you win' outcome have looked like? etc. 105

What outcome were you aiming for?

What outcome did you achieve?

How could you improve your effectiveness in achieving a win-win outcome?

The quest for excellence that drives many managers can lead them to want to win outright, and to bring everyone else into agreement with their point of view. The ability to tolerate and live with differences of opinion, and indeed to value these, is part of developing leadership effectiveness.

REFERENCES

1   Adair J. *Effective Leadership*. Pan; London. 1988.
2   Covey SR. *The seven habits of highly effective people*. Simon and Schuster; London. 1999.

"When we are 'stuck' in our thinking – whether trying to solve a problem, redesign a process, develop a new service, or delight a customer – it may not do any good to simply think harder."

Paul Plsek

Decision-making and problem-solving

Introduction

As a leader, people will look to you to make decisions on a frequent basis. Sometimes this may be straightforward, if you can draw on your own experience and knowledge to decide about an issue, and if the best solution seems clear to you. Increasingly, as your management role expands and your area of responsibility widens, you are likely to find yourself being asked to decide on issues about which you are unfamiliar, for which there does not appear to be an obvious solution, or where there are many conflicting factors to balance.

Making decisions is often linked to solving problems and this chapter considers both areas. There is an overview of why decision-making can be complex and challenging, followed by suggested approaches which can help navigate the maze of solving problems and making decision. The chapter includes systematic and more creative approaches, plus a consideration of how other people can be involved in these processes.

Information for decision-making

One of the most difficult parts of developing your leadership role is the lack of information on which decisions can be based. Managers with clinical, functional or technical backgrounds often struggle to feel confident about decisions they have made, because they do not feel that they have enough relevant information on which to base a judgement. This is understandable, given that their professional training probably centred on using sound information to inform decisions.

The process of making management decisions does not differ greatly from this. The difference is that the overlap between useful and required information is often narrow, as illustrated below. You are likely to have masses of information available, of which only some is required. And you may find that there is information you need that is not readily available.

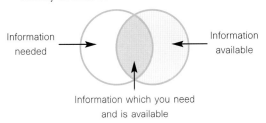

Information needed → ← Information available

Information which you need and is available

Logical decision-making

There are tried and tested models to support decision-making, which break the process down into stages as follows:

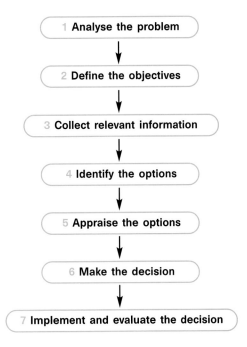

1 **Analyse the problem**

↓

2 **Define the objectives**

↓

3 **Collect relevant information**

↓

4 **Identify the options**

↓

5 **Appraise the options**

↓

6 **Make the decision**

↓

7 **Implement and evaluate the decision**

Analyse the problem: Ensure that you and those involved are clear what the issue is that you are attempting to decide on. For example, is the issue requiring action a cause of the situation or a symptom?

Define the objectives: What is the desired outcome of making this decision? It is important to be clear about this so that those involved can judge when this has been achieved and also so that expectations can be realistic.

Collect relevant information: As discussed above, it can be difficult to obtain all the relevant information and there are likely to be 'unknown' factors. Information and data need to underpin any decision, and will help to complete each of the other steps in the process.

Identify the options: Even if there are options which appear unfavourable at first, it is important to identify them, in order to avoid overlooking any possible ways to approach the situation. It also avoids the trap of jumping too quickly to 'either-or' thinking, which can limit the scope for creative options.

Appraise the options: Compare the options directly with one another on the basis of important factors, such as cost, time, and repercussions.

Make the decision: At this stage in the process, the skill is in balancing the need to strive for the best possible outcome with the requirement to finally decide. As well as managing this balance for yourself, you are likely to need to convince others of why the final decision needs to be made and possibly to persuade people to support (or at least, agree not to obstruct) the decision. It is easy to underestimate how much time and effort this stage can take, but remember that communicating with others about the decision requires careful thought and as much time as possible.

Implement and evaluate: Where action begins, arising out of the decision, and where the 'point of no return' is crossed. This is the point at which it would take more time and effort and cause more problems to go back on the decision than to move forward with it, even if you know it to be less than ideal. In your constant drive to excel and improve as a leader, the decision-making process can provide rich material to review, in order to consider how you would do things differently next time – as there is bound to be a next time.

The advantage of such a rational approach is that it provides a structured framework for working through decisions and it can bring a sense of clarity and robustness to the process. However, many decisions and problems are highly complex and do not always lend themselves well to a linear, step-by-step approach. In these cases, it is useful to be able to draw on alternative strategies for solving problems and making decisions, to complement the more logical approach.

A model for option appraisal is provided on the CD-ROM

Creative problem - solving

The essence of creative approaches to problem-solving and decision-making is in freeing the mind from the usual 'norms' of thought which dominate our interpretation of the world. This takes some practice, and people can need reassurance and encouragement that this is a legitimate approach to tackling real issues in the workplace.

As a society, our tendency is often to judge people on the extent to which their ideas correspond with those of the majority, so it requires courage to express views and ideas that may initially appear 'off the wall'. Increasingly, difficult issues at work appear intractable when they are considered in the

context of previous problem-solving approaches. So an alternative way of thinking about issues can help to 'unblock' problematic situations.

Activity 1

Try to connect up the dots in this pattern by drawing four straight lines, without taking your pencil off the page

Check your solution to this problem by looking at the answer in Appendix C.

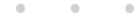

Adapted from Adair, 1997[2]

Tip: If you are struggling try to 'think outside the box'!

Problem-solving by putting yourself in the place of others

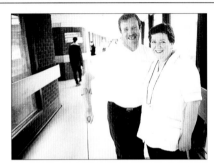

 After a year as the director of nursing, I felt there was quite a lot about the trust I had not picked up. As a nurse sitting at board level, being able to draw on recent clinical experience is very powerful. So I decided to go back to the coal face. The aim was to get out of the ivory tower my leadership role had provided. I wanted people to see me and work out my values from what I said and what I did, and I could see a bit of what life was like for them.

Over four months I have undertaken seven clinical day placements working as an auxiliary nurse in the trust. I worked in medicine, surgery and accident and emergency.

I am now much more focused on how I am going to spend the nurse education budget – on leadership training for nurses in charge and training in empowerment for healthcare assistants.

As a director on a clinical placement, you will find there are things that could be done within the resources that are available but of which middle managers are unaware. I see my role as a leader to be about empowering my staff, making sure managers have the information they need in order to help themselves. It is very important not to come in like a fairy godmother, spreading gifts. The success should belong to them.

Clinical placements are not inspections and you must judge very carefully what you do with what you see and hear. It is more important to respond to what is good and make sure people know that you have noticed.

I learned a lot about how communication systems between leaders and staff do or do not work. I don't think I treat my staff any differently now, if anything the difference is in the way they treat me. I am no longer seen as an inaccessible leader and this means I have more confidence about speaking to them informally.

Staff who wonder where the managers are just don't realise how intimidating it is to walk up to highly confident busy professionals and interrupt their work. I sometimes felt that I was 'in the way' in clinical areas.

June Andrews, director of nursing, Forth Valley Acute Hospitals trust, Falkirk

Photo: Stephen Tasker

Unlike the nine dots puzzle on page 111, most problems at work do not have one solution which is clearly the right answer. Instead, a range of possible options may be open, all of which have their pro's and cons, but none of which is completely ideal. However, the nine dots activity does remind us that at times,

'thinking outside the box' can help in generating new ways of thinking about problems and identifying possible solutions. 111

See CD-ROM for information on problem-solving styles, and a questionnaire to help you identify your own style

Lateral thinking

Edward de Bono was the originator of the phrase 'lateral thinking', which means thinking to the sides, looking across and around rather than thinking vertically, and looking up and down.

It can take practise to think laterally, as it often involves deliberately avoiding the logical or 'automatic' way of doing things, and challenging the assumptions we make about issues or problems.

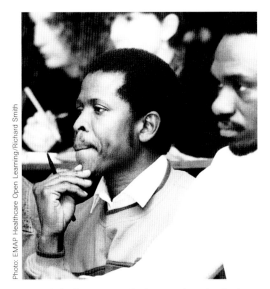

Photo: EMAP Healthcare Open Learning/Richard Smith

Lateral thinking means thinking to the sides, looking across and around rather than thinking vertically.

Vertical thinking	Lateral thinking
• Looks for what is right • Concentrates on relevance • Moves in the most likely directions • One thing must follow directly from another	• Looks for what is different • Welcomes chance intrusions • Explores the least likely directions • Makes deliberate jumps **Adapted from Adair, 1997[2]**

De Bono's six thinking hats

White hat thinking

This covers facts, figures, information needs and gaps. 'I think we need some white hat thinking at this point...' means 'let's drop the arguments and proposals, and look at the data'.

Red hat thinking

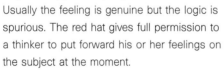

This covers intuition, feelings and emotions. The red hat allows the thinker to put forward an intuition without any need to justify it. 'Putting on my red hat, I think this is a terrible proposal.' Usually, feelings and intuition can only be introduced into a discussion if they are supported by logic. Usually the feeling is genuine but the logic is spurious. The red hat gives full permission to a thinker to put forward his or her feelings on the subject at the moment.

Black hat thinking

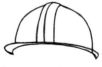

This is the hat of judgement and caution. It is a most valuable hat. It is not in any sense an inferior or negative hat. The black hat is used to point out why a suggestion does not fit the facts, the available experience, the system in use, or the policy that is being followed. The black hat must always be logical.

Yellow hat thinking

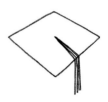

This is the logical and positive hat. Why something will work and why it will offer benefits. It can be used in looking forward to the results of some proposed action, but can also be used to find something of value in what has already happened.

Green hat thinking

This is the hat of creativity, alternatives, proposals, what is interesting, provocations and changes.

Blue hat thinking

This is the overview or process control hat, which brings structure and order to the thinking process. It looks not at the subject itself but at the 'thinking' about the subject. 'Putting on my blue hat, I feel we should do some more green hat thinking at this point.'

From Edward de Bono's *Why do quality efforts lose their fizz?*[3]

De Bono developed the idea of six different ways of thinking, represented by his 'six thinking hats'. There are six metaphorical hats and the thinker can put on or take off one of these hats to indicate the type of thinking being used.

The benefit of using the six thinking hats approach is that the hat becomes the thinking style of the person 'wearing' it, regardless of whether this is their natural style or not. It both encourages people to try out new thinking styles and removes any focus from people whose usual thinking style is more or less helpful. When done in a group situation, everybody 'wears' the same hat at the same time.

Activity 2

Think about a problem you have at work and jot down the options you think you have for tackling the problem.

For each option in turn, adopt the style of thinking of each of De Bono's six thinking hats.

How does each hat change the way you look at the problem?

Creative thinking

'If you always do what you always did, you always get what you always got.'

Mark Twain

A natural way to approach decisions and to solve problems is to use previous experience as a reference point in assessing the current situation. Writers such as Paul Plsek reject this approach, arguing that relying on memory of past incidents and problems stimulates automatic responses based on previous approaches.[1] The result is the same sort of solutions as in the past, rather than new ideas for overcoming problems.

For creative thinking, the first requirement is to resist turning to our previous experience for answers, but instead to consciously challenge our usual responses and to focus instead on the things we would normally pay least attention to. This involves escaping from current ways of thinking, breaking out of usual rules and boundaries and even thinking beyond the actual place and time. From this, it is then easier to move towards another point of view.

This is the basis for Plsek's approach to creative thinking, which is known as 'directed creativity'. Plsek's definition of directed creativity is 'the purposeful production of creative ideas in a topic area, followed up by deliberate effort to implement some of those ideas'. In other words, it is the use of creative thinking principles in a focused way, with the intention of putting the emerging ideas into practice in reality.

Activity 3

Use some of the creative thinking techniques on the CD-ROM to think through a problem you have at work.

Make a note of:

1 What are the assumptions you automatically make about the situation?

2 What would be your approach to the situation based on past experience?

3 What rules and boundaries can you escape from if you start to think more creatively?

4 What new ideas emerge when you try out some of Plsek's suggested directed creativity techniques?

See the CD-ROM for some tools and techniques based on Plsek's directed creativity approach

Brainstorming

One of the most popular techniques for creative thinking is brainstorming. This is a tool that is quick, inclusive, informal and when used properly can generate good ideas.

The principle behind this approach is to create an environment where people are permitted and encouraged to 'think out of the box', come up with unusual ideas and let their imagination run free. Analysing and judging ideas do not form part of brainstorming; the purpose is purely to identify as many options as possible.

Involving others in decision-making

As a leader, there is more to making a decision than merely deciding for yourself on the best way forward. Others may disagree with you, and it is likely that they

Creative problem-solving at work

An ambulance trust wanted to prevent the ambulance crew missing their meal-breaks or having these interrupted. The chief executive introduced a compensation scheme which paid £5 to each crew member who had a missed or interrupted mealbreak. The crew now don't know whether they want a peaceful mealbreak or not.

A cardiac unit with a shortage of physiotherapists has trained up healthcare assistants to undertake post-stroke therapy treatments to free up physiotherapy time.

will be key to implementing what you have decided, so gaining their commitment is a central part of making a decision. This means involving your team and others affected in each stage of the decision-making process, from clarifying what the aim is to implementing and evaluating the outcome.

It is often easy to assume that because you have been closely involved with sorting out a problem or making a decision, other people are equally aware of the issues involved. It is worth taking the time to involve people in decisions from the very beginning, so that once the final decision is made, you can be confident that others understand how and why this was arrived at.

Some people will choose not to engage in the decision-making process and are willing to let

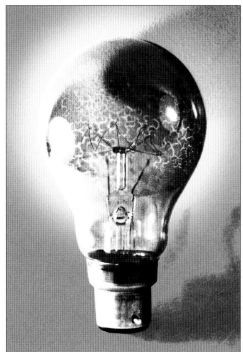

Photo: Rhiannon Frost

Brainstorming should create an environment where people can come up with unusual ideas and let their imaginations run free.

Guidelines for brainstorming	
Clarify the question	Make it clear what the brainstorming ideas are intended for, eg – 'How can we reduce the 'Did Not Attend' rate?' or 'What could we bid for from the modernisation fund?'
Suspend judgement	Put all ideas onto a flipchart as 'raw material', without starting to consider whether they will work. There is no such thing as a 'silly idea' at this stage.
Avoid detail	Just capture the essence of the idea, without looking for lots of detail.
Encourage creativity	The more unusual the ideas, the better. Encourage people to let their minds run free.
Go for quality	When ideas appear to have dried up, don't curtail the brainstorming straight away – try to aim for as many ideas as possible.
Take a (short) break	After the initial flood of ideas, build in a two minute discussion of something unrelated and light, such as a soap opera or holiday destinations. This allows people to continue to think about the main issue whilst filling time with easy conversation, and can generate another range of ideas.
Build on ideas	Encourage people to extend and build on the ideas of others.

others make the decisions. Others will resist taking part because they fear the outcome or they object to the process. People will ultimately make their own choices about these things, but as a leader it is your role to find ways of enabling people to be involved and to persuade and influence them about the merits of contributing to solving problems and making decisions.

Activity 4

Think of a decision you recently made which affects other people. List up to eight key people affected by the decision, but who were not necessarily involved in the decision making process. For each person listed, imagine how the decision appears to them (ie, see it through their eyes)

Do they know:

- Why the decision was reached?
- What other options were considered?
- How the decision will affect them?
- Who was involved in making the decision?

What could you do next time to increase the involvement and awareness of others in the decision-making process?

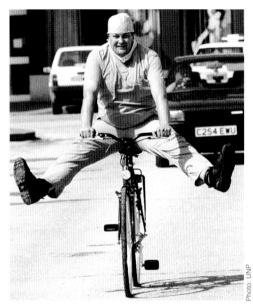

Incorporating short breaks or 'playtime' activities like cycling into your creative thinking sessions can be rewarding and help stimulate fresh thought.

Other creative thinking techniques

There are lots of different techniques for creative thinking. Here are a few more you can try.

- **Imitating ideas:** There is no need to constantly re-invent the wheel. Think about how similar problems to yours have been solved by other industries and then consider whether you might be able to adapt their solution to your problem. For example, the NHS has already taken its lead from the airline industry in starting to implement patient booking schemes. What else can you adapt?

- Role playing: Not everyone likes role playing, but it can be an invaluable tool in helping you to look at problems from a different perspective. For example, put yourself in the place of patients accessing your service and then ask questions like: how does the service appear to them? why are they using it? how would they see the problem? what solution would they like to see?

- Blue sky thinking: By dreaming of your ideal situation or solution, you can often come up with new and workable ideas. Allow your imagination to roam free. Ask questions like: what would my perfect situation be? What impact would this have? What would I do if I have unlimited resources? etc.

Barriers to creative thinking

There are a number of factors that you will need to take into consideration when employing creative thinking techniques. You may find that you encounter obstruction for the following reasons:

- Fear – people often feel threatened if you try to introduce new ways of doing things. Think about how you would deal with this.

- If it ain't broke, don't fix it. Explain that it is always worth looking at how systems operate now because there might be still better ways of doing things.

- Time – busy people won't always see this as a necessity. Make sure you give plenty of notice so that people can plan their workloads accordingly.

- Lack of practice and the techniques you use. For creative thinking to work properly, you need to know what you are doing. Make sure you are confident about the tools you will be using and your aims before you embark on the process.

- The type of people. You will often need to convince people of the value of creative thinking. Explain that using creative thinking techniques to solve problems can also frequently result in a better service to patients, savings in both monetary and time terms, an improvement in quality, etc.

• SWOT analysis: A SWOT analysis allows you to examine your strengths, weaknesses, opportunities and threats. It is a good way of looking at what you do well now, what you do badly and what can be improved, what chances and trends are facing you and what obstacles you are facing. Carrying out this analysis will often be illuminating – both in terms of pointing out what needs to be done, and in putting problems into perspective.

Borrowing ideas from industry

 KPMG in the Netherlands had identified problems with their structure which held them back as a company. The company needed to change its culture. As part of the process they held creative events designed to tease out new ideas. They pulled together 100 people at an Oprah Winfrey-style meeting in a large auditorium; they developed a 'yellow card' system to flag up old, inappropriate workplace behaviours; they produced objects to symbolise the new culture. They held 'playtime' events including bike rides and laser gun fights at the local amusement centre. All these events helped create an understanding of the company's present culture, of the culture they would like to shift towards and how to go about it.

Source: *Leadership and management excellence; corporate development strategies,* 2001[3]

REFERENCES

1   Plsek PE. *Creativity, innovation and quality.* ASQC Quality Press,1997.

2   De Bono E. *'Why do quality efforts lose their fizz?' Quality is no longer enough.* The Journal for Quality and Participation, September 1991.

3   James K. *Leadership and management excellence; corporate development strategies.* London; Council for Excellence in Management and Leadership, 2001.

Notes

"Stress occurs when pressure exceeds your perceived ability to cope."

Cooper and Palmer

Managing stress

Introduction

We often talk about stress as something related to external pressure, such as lack of time or certain demanding situations. However, researchers in the field emphasise that stress arises from a combination of internal and external factors. This definition acknowledges the role of external 'pressure' whilst highlighting that a person's attitude to coping with pressure determines the extent of their stress.

As a leader, manager or practitioner, work is often demanding and pressurised, and it is a real challenge to effectively balance the competing demands. In addition, it is important to acknowledge that one of the single most frequently quoted reasons for workplace stress is poor management and a lack of leadership.

This chapter provides an overview of some of the current thinking on stress management, and provides practical suggestions of how you can identify what triggers stress for you and take action to deal with them more effectively.

Identifying stress

Dr Cary Cooper is a writer and researcher in stress management, and maintains that a large part of a person's stress is related to their own expectations and beliefs. If a person has a set of strong convictions about how they and others should and ought to behave, then they are more likely to become stressed when things go wrong than people who have more moderate beliefs.

Look at the list of beliefs on page 126. If you hold any of these beliefs strongly, then when things don't go according to plan, stress may result. If you hold 10 or more of these beliefs strongly, then it is likely that your own beliefs contribute greatly to your stress levels. Even when these beliefs are held moderately, they can turn many situations into potentially stressful events. **126**

The following thought patterns based on certain beliefs have been shown to contribute to stress and act as an obstacle to dealing effectively with stress.

All-or-nothing thinking: Viewing things in absolute or extreme terms, black and white,

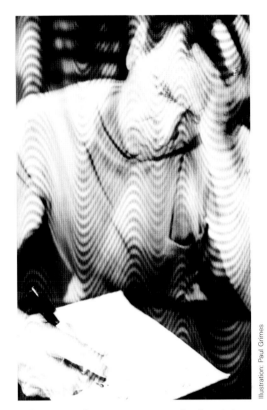

A large part of a person's stress is related to their own expectations and beliefs.

Illustration: Paul Grimes

with no shade of grey. Eg – a job is only worth doing if it is done properly.

Labelling: We attach a universal label to ourselves and others. Eg – they're late again. That's another sign that they're totally incompetent.

				Stress inducing beliefs indicator

Stress inducing beliefs indicator

The questions that follow include both work and general beliefs.

Put a circle around the strength of your belief:

S = strongly   **M**= moderately   **W**= weakly

Include in question 25 any additional beliefs you hold that cause you further stress.

1	S	M	W	Events should go smoothly
2	S	M	W	Work must be exciting and stimulating
3	S	M	W	If I lost my job, life would be awful
4	S	M	W	If I lost my job, I couldn't bear it
5	S	M	W	My job is one of the most important things to me
6	S	M	W	I must perform well at all important tasks
7	S	M	W	My work should be recognised by others
8	S	M	W	I am indispensable at work
9	S	M	W	I must enjoy myself whatever I'm doing
10	S	M	W	I must not get bored
11	S	M	W	I should not encounter problems
12	S	M	W	I should have the solitude I deserve
13	S	M	W	I must escape from responsibilities and demands
14	S	M	W	I should be treated fairly
15	S	M	W	I should be treated as special
16	S	M	W	I should be in control of all significant situations
17	S	M	W	Others should respect me
18	S	M	W	I should get on well with my friends and family
19	S	M	W	My children should do well in life
20	S	M	W	If things went badly, it would be awful
21	S	M	W	If things went badly, I couldn't stand it
22	S	M	W	Things never work out well for me
23	S	M	W	If things go wrong, those responsible are 'useless', 'idiots' or 'failures'
25	S	M	W	If I fail at a task, it proves I'm a failure
25	S	M	W	Additional beliefs ....

Source: C Cooper and S Palmer *Conquer your Stress*, 2000

Negative focus: The tendency to only focus on the negative aspects of things. Eg – things are always going wrong in my job.

Discounting the positive: Interpreting anything positive as unimportant or insignificant. Eg – when my manager praises me, they are only doing it to be nice; they don't really mean it.

Mind-reading: Assuming that people's behaviour means they are thinking negatively about you. Eg – they haven't spoken to me all morning – I must have done something to upset them.

Fortune-telling: Predicting the worst without evidence to support this. Eg – what's the point of saying anything? They are bound to disagree with me.

Magnification: Attributing more significance to a negative event than is warranted. Eg – if this presentation goes badly, it will be the end of my career

Minimisation: Making excuses for our successes and condemning our shortcomings. Eg – I was just lucky to get the job – in the right place at the right time.

Blame: Blaming others for problems rather than taking any personal responsibility. Eg – it's not surprising I made a mistake: they have given me far too much to do.

Personalisation: Blaming ourselves unfairly for something for which we are not completely responsible. Eg – my staff did not reach the target. It's all my fault.

Being over-demanding: Holding unrealistic expectations or rigid beliefs expressed as 'should', 'must', 'got to', 'have to ' and 'ought'. Eg – I must always perform well despite my worries.

Phoney-ism: Fearing that others may find out we are not the person we portray. Eg – one day I'll make a mistake and they'll find out that I'm not up to the job.

Activity 1

Think about a current or recent problem, which caused you to feel stressed. Go through the list of thought patterns listed on p125-127, and note what you were thinking under any of these categories that seem applicable. Consider also the beliefs that you marked as 'strong' in the stress inducing beliefs Indicator on page 126 and think about how these affected your response to your problem. 125

A model of stress

The importance of beliefs is also central to Dr Albert Ellis' ABC model of stress:

A Activating event or situation

B Beliefs about the event

C Consequences: emotional (eg – anxiety)
behavioural (eg – aggression)
physiological (eg – palpitations)

In order to help people deal with C, the consequences of stress, there are a further two stages to the model:

D Disputing the beliefs at 'B'

E Effectively dealing with the activating events 'A'.

If we can identify our beliefs at B, and the thought patterns which accompany these, it is possible to start to challenge and dispute these at 'D', in order to develop new ways of thinking about situations. This helps to create a more effective approach to dealing with stress.

Strategies for handling stress

Our beliefs are deeply-rooted and it is unrealistic to expect these to change overnight. However, with time and concentrated effort, it is possible to alter the way we look at situations in order to reduce the negative impact which stressful events can have. This does not mean changing your whole value base or radically transforming your attitudes. Rather, it involves considering that there are alternative ways of thinking about situations, and reviewing how your own thoughts and views can help rather than hinder you in dealing with stressful situations.

Life at work and home is often riddled with difficulties, and these factors are often

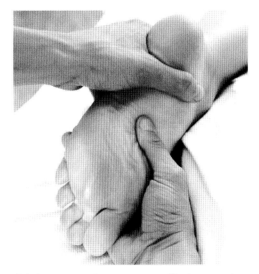

It is important to have your own effective strategies for dealing with personal stress in order that you can support others in coping with day-to-day demands.

beyond our control. What is within our sphere of influence is our own response to events. Becoming more aware of how difficult situations affect you and your thinking is the first step to more handling stress more effectively.

It can be tempting to get into the habit of working long hours as a way of keeping up with the demands of the job. However, evidence strongly suggests that this is not an effective response to work pressure. As a leader, it is vital to realise that much of your

behaviour sets an example to other members of staff. You will be more effective and more motivated if you take your annual leave entitlement and ensure you limit your working week to a reasonable number of hours.

The *Improving Working Lives* policy requirements in the NHS means that organisations are required to find ways of making working practices more flexible for employees. Underpinning this guidance is the acknowledgement that a healthy work-life balance should be achievable for all staff.

As a leader, it is important to have your own effective strategies for dealing with personal stress in order that you can support others in coping with day-to-day demands, too. A tired, frazzled leader will not be much use to anyone.

See the CD-ROM for examples of strategies for adapting the way you think about stressful events

REFERENCES

1   Cooper CL, Palmer S. *Conquer your stress* Chartered Institute of Personnel Development; Management Shapers Series, 2000.

Notes

"The axiom for today's change leaders should be: don't plan but be prepared. People who make rigid plans are all too often the ones who are least adequately prepared."

Charles Handy [1]

Leadership into the future

Introduction

In his book *The age of unreason* Charles Handy tells the story of a frog being slowly heated in a pan of water. As the temperature rises, the frog feels increasingly uncomfortable, but because the change is very gradual, the frog remains in the water until it is ultimately boiled alive. If the frog had been plunged into the very hot water initially, it would have jumped straight out in shock, but because the water very slowly became hotter, the frog failed to respond to the gradual changes which threatened it.[1]

This tale illustrates how important it is to anticipate change and to be constantly looking at what gradual and small changes mean in the 'bigger picture'. This chapter considers the leader's role in the process of 'horizon-scanning'. It also suggests ways in which you can keep abreast of the rapid and constantly evolving environment, in order to help you become more prepared for change.

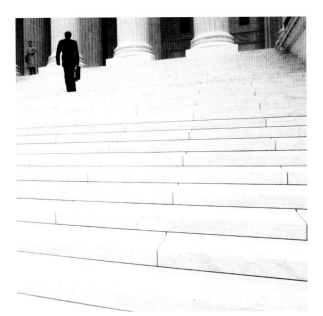

Leaders play a key role in shaping a vision of where the future might lie.

Leading into the future

Leadership involves making sense of internal and external trends, changes, developments and pressures and understanding the possible impact of these on the future. Leaders play a key role in shaping a vision of where the future might lie and providing a sense of direction of how to move positively forward.

Of course, nobody can know for certain what the future holds. Uncertainty about the future can be damaging and unsettling for all involved, and one of the key ways in which leaders add value to their teams and organisations is by helping to provide a positive approach to identifying and shaping the future. This includes communicating the vision and supporting others in being prepared for change.

Scanning the horizon

Public and private sector organisations continually face new pressures to adapt, learn, innovate and keep up with changes in the external environment and in society generally. Amongst these new pressures are:

- Rapid technological developments.
- Innovations in telecommunications.
- More complex, fluid organisational forms and structures, designed to be more flexible, responsive and able to adapt to change quickly.
- Increased consumer expectations of service delivery. (See box on page 134)
- Changing attitudes to work and lifestyle.
- Changing demographics.
- 'Globalisation' of many sectors, meaning increased international focus.

Articulating the vision: Communicating a clear vision for the whole health community

What do good leaders do?	What does this mean in practice?
Leaders show that they have a clear picture of the world they aspire to create and build upon. They also have a positive sense of how their vision accords with that of peers and of the organisation as a whole. Nor is their vision narrowly confined to the organisation: it takes in a wider perspective, showing how the organisation contributes to creating the future.	• Having an adequate rationale for the vision. • Demonstrating that they are in touch with current reality. • Showing how the vision can be realised. • Engaging people in developing the vision and making it more tangible. • Relating the vision to individual values, beliefs and concerns.
Leaders are able to show why their vision is worth striving for and how it can be brought into reality. In articulating their vision, leaders show that they are in touch with current reality but demonstrate that the new vision is attainable. They relate it to the diversity of values, beliefs and concerns of the people, groups and communities they communicate with. In doing so, they engender a sense of excitement and confidence in people's ability to achieve something worthwhile.	• Relating the vision to that of peers and of the wider health community and beyond. • Making adequate time to communicate and discuss the vision. • Conveying the vision with passion and conviction. • Listening to and acknowledging concerns and alternative viewpoints. • Reflecting in the vision the diversity of the communities they serve. • Engendering confidence and belief in the vision and people's ability to achieve it.

Source: *Workforce and Development: Embodying leadership in the NHS, 2000*[2]

Rising public expectations

People expect from public services the standards which they themselves are expected to provide in their own jobs. They expect service of the kind which they would get from the private sector.

Sir Richard Wilson, Cabinet Secretary

Source: Performance and Innovation Unit, 2000[3]

Activity 1

Think back five years and note down some of the key changes that have happened since then under the following headings:

- Social, eg – more elderly people requiring care, fewer people choosing to work in certain parts of the public sector.
- Technological, eg – development of non-invasive treatment techniques, e-mail, the Internet.
- Environmental, eg – creation of new housing estates, building of new transport links.
- Political, eg – outcomes of general or local elections, changes to NHS structure.

What difference have these changes made to your service area(s)?

What trends do you expect to see over the next five years under each these headings?

What will be the impact of these trends on your service area?

Some of the factors are unique to public services. These include:

- A focus on addressing cross-cutting issues, such as social exclusion.

- Increased pressure for seamless, personalised services, across public, private and voluntary sectors to ensure that services meet the needs of the user.

- Greater pressures for continuous improvement, innovation and learning.

- A more complex political and institutional context, including devolved government, local and regional bodies and the European Union.

Being prepared for change

The theory of change management has a long history of developing models moving organisations and people from one set of circumstances to another, from A to B, overcoming resistance along the way. In Chapter one, we considered the way in which transformational styles of management have evolved, in response to rapid and continuous changes, and the need for much more flexible and nimble organisations. ←5

In line with these developments, there has been an emphasis in the NHS on transformational models of leadership, and

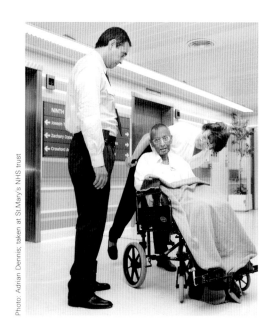

Ara Darzi and Eve Knight, members of the Modernisation Board, went 'back to the shop floor' to gain insight into the experiences of those actively providing health services.

accompanying this, an increasing interest in the organisation development approach to change. The emphasis of this approach is less about 'changing an organisation', and much more linked to creating 'a changing organisation'. Key features of the approach are accepting the continuous nature of change and designing the organisation and its systems in a way that enables it to adapt quickly and proactively to future directions. A key part of this is also about supporting staff to take a positive and proactive approach to change.

As a leader in an increasingly complex healthcare environment, you have your own part to play in developing this sort of organisation – or at least in your area of the

Readiness for change

Except for only the most extreme situations, all change in human systems is ultimately voluntary. Forcing the spread of a change onto a largely unwilling organisation builds resentment that makes that change, and all future change, hard to accomplish. If readiness is not high, take time to build it. Relative to the ultimate goal of spreading the change, this seeming delay is a better use of time than succumbing to pressure to roll out the change against the tide of lack of awareness of the need, apathy, or outright opposition. At the same time, keep in mind that you may only need readiness in a portion of the target population in order to reach the tipping point where the idea begins to spread quickly on its own.

Paul Plsek, 2000[4]

organisation. The final section of this book explores some of the ways in which you can keep abreast of the changes and developments affecting your area of work, in order that you are better prepared to lead positively into the future. Awareness of the elements described below will help you to plan how you can keep abreast of the rapidly changing environment.

Learning from overseas and industry

Many of the service improvement initiatives evident in the NHS have evolved from original approaches in other countries, most notably from the USA and from Japan.

Change management approaches such as total quality management and business process re-engineering are examples of initiatives that have been adapted and applied to healthcare settings in Britain, having originated overseas. TQM drew on experience in manufacturing industry in Japan and was prominent in the UK during the 1980s, focusing on replicating Japanese success in achieving high levels of productivity at the same time as achieving or exceeding customer expectations.

Business process re-engineering is another example of an approach to change which was adapted from industry overseas, and in the case of the NHS, focused on starting from scratch and redesigning the patient pathway from one which is convenient to the system to one which is centred on the patient.

The NHS modernisation agenda has placed at its heart several approaches to service improvement, based on ideas and concepts from overseas and from industry. These have recently been grouped together under the NHS Modernisation Agency and include:

- **Process redesign** – mapping the patient process from beginning to end to identify how it can be improved.

- **Booked admissions** – an approach which aims for patients to be given a date for their appointment or admission at the time the decision is made to refer or admit, based on what is convenient to them.

- **Diagnostic and treatment centres** – a new way of delivering elective care, which moves almost all elective work out of acute hospitals and into dedicated units. This is intended to avoid emergency work interrrupting booked and planned elective care.

- **'Collaboratives'** – influenced by the work of Don Berwick, Director of the US Institute for Healthcare Improvement. Berwick's approach to quality improvement emphasises that mistakes and delays in care are usually to do with the systems and processes of care, which have become institutionalised, rather than merely due to individual error. Collaboratives have so far been implemented in orthopaedics, cancer care, primary care, coronary heart disease and in-patient mental health. They bring together groups of 20-40 healthcare organisations in a mutual support and learning network to focus on improving a specific clinical or operational area.

These examples illustrate that there is much to be learnt from how other industries and countries approach change and improvement processes. Leadership is at the heart of the success of all the approaches described, as they rely primarily on the co-operation of clinical teams.

Keeping abreast of developments

Networks

Organised networks are increasingly proving to be popular and effective vehicles for sharing and exploring changes, developments and new approaches in health and many other sectors. Usually, a network will focus on a specific area of interest, and will attract people who are concerned with this to join together, pool resources, gather and share ideas and consider the future for their area of interest. Many networks are supplemented by websites, e-mail discussion forums and electronic library resources. Networks can help leaders and managers to broaden their view of their particular field of work, and look beyond their immediate organisation or environment.

Clinical networks have also developed rapidly in recent years. These recognise that clinical specialties cross organisational and geographic boundaries, and that there is benefit in sharing and learning within a clinical specialty. Clinical networks also aim to avoid duplication of effort and resources. The development of cancer networks are now a requirement of health communities, and many others are being developed.

NHS Learning Network

The NHS Learning Network was established to support the process of modernisation in health services, and as a resource for managers and practitioners alike. It focuses on pooling and sharing knowledge and information about effective approaches to improving services, and the network provides several practical ways:

- Learning centres and learning partnerships – NHS organisations which lead in providing opportunities for people to learn from one another about changes and effective ways of responding to these.

- Management and leadership development.

- Providing information and evidence to help NHS staff learn about service developments.

See http://www.doh.gov.uk/learningzone/ best_pra.htm for more details on the NHS Learning Network and its related activities and resources

Databases

The rapid development of information systems means that accessing up-to-date information is easier and quicker than ever before. Many databases have been created, which contain research findings and sources of literature to support decision-making, as well as examples of good practice from elsewhere in the NHS.

An example is the Service Delivery Practice database. The principal purpose of the database is to enable the sharing of information between NHS individuals and organisations to improve service delivery. This is achieved by the sharing of information about projects, complete or not, successful or not, in a safe and non-judgmental way, on the internal NHSweb. This enables others to see what is being done, to learn from the experience of service colleagues, and to comment on the activities shown. There is also the opportunity to place details of successful initiatives onto the database, for others to learn from.

See http://www.doh.gov.uk/learningzone/ sdpinter.htm for more information

Beacons

The NHS Beacon programme was launched in 1999 as a way of encouraging NHS organisations to share good practice. 'Beacon sites' can be a useful reference point for understanding how others have responded to some of the changes in your sector. Visits and workshops are organised by beacon sites, to share their innovations with people from other parts of the health sector. Details of beacon sites are available in an annual guidebook and from the NHS Beacons website. (See Further reading list.) 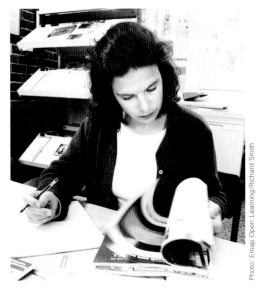143

Management and clinical journals

Journals and periodicals provide a highly accessible way of keeping abreast of developments in a particular field. There are numerous journals within every clinical specialty, as well as more general publications which focus on issues related to healthcare organisations and management. The library at your local NHS trust, or within the healthcare faculty of your local university is a good place to start to find these. See also the list of useful websites in the section on Further reading. 143

Journals and periodicals provide a highly accessible way of keeping abreast of developments in a particular field.

Conferences and seminars

Many of the professional institutes, such as the Institute of Healthcare Management and the NHS Confederation, organise annual conferences. These are a chance to hear practitioners, policy-makers and politicians outline the latest developments in healthcare, and to attend workshops which provide a chance to explore issues in more detail.

Organisations such as the King's Fund and the Health Services Management Centre in

Birmingham run seminars to disseminate thinking and research in the latest policy areas.

Leading change

The scope to explore new developments and trends is almost limitless, and it has never been easier for leaders in the health sector to access knowledge and information about trends and changes. The difficulty can lie in identifying just what you need to know when so much information is available.

Previous sections of this book have underlined the importance of keeping abreast of changes in order to lead services and colleagues forward and to continually improve health and healthcare. Everyone has their own strategies and approach to keeping up-to-date. A first step in becoming an effective leader is to decide:

How will I keep abreast of changes and developments:

- In the rest of the world?
- In other sectors of health and social care?
- In my own sector across the country?
- Within my own organisation?

Developing your own strategies and plans for keeping up-to-date is the first step in developing your ability to lead change. Choose approaches which suit your learning style, stimulate your personal and professional interests, and which fit in with your working patterns. Aim to build these processes in to your day-to-day work,

Activity 2

Imagine it is now the year 2007. From what you know of current trends and developments, write down some of the changes you would expect to see in your service area(s) between now and then. Highlight whether these are a result of social, technological, environmental, political or other factors.

What evidence do you have to suggest that these changes are likely?

What would need to be done to ensure that your service area(s) approaches these changes positively?

Identify steps you can personally take:

a) To help identify where the future of your service area lies, and

b) To support and prepare others for the changes and developments which lie ahead.

making links between the changing
environment and your area of practice, and
share your discoveries with others.

As you become more aware of the 'shifting
sands' in which the health sector operates, the
future may look more uncertain than you
anticipated. But your growing awareness is
likely to bring with it deeper insight into the
possibilities of the future – possibilities for
patients, for your services and for those
whom you lead.

REFERENCES

1   Handy C. *The age of unreason.* Arrow Business
    Books, London. 1995.

2   Workforce and development leadership working
    group. *Workforce and development: Embodying
    leadership in the NHS.* London; NHS Executive, 2000.

3   Performance and Innovation Unit. *Strengthening
    leadership in the public sector.* (See
    http://www.cabinet-office.gov.uk/innovation) 2000.

4   Plsek P. *Spreading good ideas for better healthcare
    – A practical toolkit.* VHA 2000 Research Series
    TX. 2000.

Further reading

Chapter one – What is leadership?

Adair J. *John Adair's 100 greatest leadership ideas*. Capstone Publishing, 2001.

Bass BM. *Leadership and performance beyond expectations*.
New York; Free Press, 1985.

Kotter J. *A force for change: How leadership differs from management*.
London; Free Press, 1990.

Kouzes JM, Posner BZ. *The leadership challenge*. San Francisco; Jossey-Bass, 1987.

Rosenbach WE, Taylor RL (eds). *Contemporary issues in leadership*.
Oxford; Westview Press, 1993.

Wright P. *Managerial leadership*. London; Routledge, 1996.

Career management and development

Evans C. A review of career anchors in use. *European Journal of Work and Organizational Psychology* Vol.5 No.4 1996: 609-615.

Hopson B, Scally M. *Build your own rainbow: a workbook for career and life management*. London; Management Books, 1999.

Strickland R. Career self-management - can we live without it? *European Journal of Work and Organizational Psychology* Vol.5 No.4 1996: 583-596.

Chapter two - Leadership in context

Heifetz RA. *Leadership without easy answers.* Cambridge; Belknap Press, 1994.

The learning organisation

Argyris C. Teaching smart people how to learn. *Harvard Business Review*, May – June 1991.

Garratt B. *The fish rots from the head – the crisis in our boardrooms: developing the crucial skills of the company director.* Harper Collins, 1997.

Clinical governance

Department of Health. *Clinical Governance in the NHS.* HSC 1999/065.

Dewar S. *Clinical governance under construction.* London; King's Fund, 1999.

Hallett L, Thompson M. *Clinical governance - a practical guide for managers.* London; Emap Public Sector Management, 2001.

Scott G. Accountability for service excellence. *Journal of Healthcare Management* Vol.46 (3):152-5, May-Jun. 2001.

Clutterbuck, D. E*veryone needs a mentor: fostering talent at work.*
London; Institute of Personnel Management, 1991.

360 degree appraisal and feedback

Tornow W, London M. *Maximising the value of 360 degree feedback (A process for individual and organisational development).* Centre for Creative Leadership, 1998.

The Institute of Managers produce a booklet on 'Using 360 degree feedback' (£3 or £2 for members) available from www.inst-management.org.uk

Guidelines, information and on-line resources for 360 degree appraisal are available from www.the360.co.uk and www.etsplc.com.

Networking

Alexander L. *Career networking: how to develop the right contacts to help you throughout your working life.* How to Books, 1997.

Bloch S. Networking for successful career management. *Training and Development (UK)* Vol.12 No.7 July 1994: 44,46.

Catt H, Scudamore P. *The power of networking: the power of using your contacts to advance your career.* Kogan Page, 1999.

Emotional intelligence

Goleman D. *Emotional intelligence.* Bloomsbury, 1996.

Chapter four – Developing others

Honey P. *101 ways to develop your people, without really trying.* London; Peter Honey, 1994.

Parsloe E, Wray M. *Coaching and mentoring: practical methods to improve learning.* Kogan Page, 2000.

Chapter five – Building effective teams

Adair J. *Effective teambuilding.* Gower; London, 1986.

Belbin RM. *Beyond the team.* Butterworth Heinemann, 2000.

Belbin RM. *Management teams - Why they succeed or fail.* Butterworth Heinemann, 1981.

Belbin RM. *Team roles at work.* Butterworth Heinemann, 1993.

Hardingham A, Ellis C. *Exercises for team development.* London; CIPD, 1999.

Hastings C, Bixby P, Chaudhry-Lawton R. *Superteams: Building organizational success through high-performing teams.* London; Harper Collins, 1994.

Larson C, Lafasto FMJ. Teamwork – *What must go right and what can go wrong.* London; Sage, 1989.

See the Belbin website at www.belbin.com

Tuckman B. Developmental sequence in small groups. *Psychological Bulletin*, 63, 1965: 384-389

Chapter six – Communicating and influencing

Influencing Others

Fisher R, Ury W. *Getting to yes.* Boston; Houghton Mifflin, 1981.

Honey P. *Improve your people skills.* 2nd edition. London; Institute of Personnel & Development, 1997.

Gillen T. *Positive influencing skills.* London; Institute of Personnel & Development, 1995.

Lambert T. *The power of influence*. London; Nicholas Brealey Publishing, 1995.

Chapter seven - Decision making and problem-solving

Adair J. *Effective decision making*. London; Pan, 1985.

Adair J. *Effective innovation.* London; Pan, 1996.

Adair J. *Decision making and problem solving.* London; Institute of Personnel & Development, 1997.

Buzan T. *Use your head.* London; BBC Publications, 1974.

De Bono E. *Lateral thinking for management.* Maidenhead; McGraw-Hill, 1971.

De Bono E. *Six thinking hats.* Little, Brown and Co, 1985.

Chapter eight – Managing stress

Bailey R. *Activities for managing stress.* London; Gower, 1989.

Cooper C L, Palmer S. *Conquer your stress.* Chartered Institute of Personnel and Development; Management Shapers series, 2000.

Newton T. *'Managing' stress: emotion and power at work.* London; Sage, 1995.

Chapter nine – Leadership into the future

Iles V, Sutherland K. *Organisational change – A review for healthcare managers, researchers and professionals.* London; NCCSDO, 2001.

Quigley, JV. *Vision: How leaders develop it, share it and sustain it.* New York; McGraw-Hill, 1993.

Making Informed Decisions on Change – Key points for health care managers and professionals. London; NCCSDO, 2001.

Locock, L *Maps and Journeys : Redesign in the NHS* Health Services Management Centre, University of Birmingham, 2001.

Bevan, H. Do improvement methods from industry work in healthcare? The case of The Leicester Royal Infirmary re-engineering programme (forthcoming).

DOH. *Managed Clinical Networks* South East Regional Office Briefing September, 2000.

Useful organisations

Association of Healthcare Human
Resource Management
AHHRM office
The Chapel Block
Barrow Hospital
Barrow Gurney
Bristol BS48 3SG
01275 394438 (telephone and fax)

British Association of Medical Managers
Third floor
Petersgate House
St Petersgate
Stockport SK1 1HE
0161 474 1141

Commission for Health Improvement
Finsbury Tower
103 – 105 Bunhill Row
London EC1Y 8TG
020 7448 9200

Health Service Journal
Greater London House
Hamsptead Road
London NW1
020 7874 0200

Health Services Management Centre
University of Birmingham
Park House
40 Edgbaston Road
Birmingham
B15 2RT
0121 414 7050

Institute for Healthcare Management
46-48 Grosvenor Gardens
London SW1 0EB
020 7881 9235

King's Fund
11-13 Cavendish Square
London W1M OAN
020 7307 2400

NHS Confederation
1 Warwick Row
London SW1E 5ER
020 7959 7272

NHS Modernisation Agency
Richmond House
79 Whitehall
London SW1 2NS

Appendix A — About the CD-ROM

The CD-ROM included with *Leadership at every level – a practical guide for managers* contains a range of useful tools and related reading materials. When using the book, you will frequently encounter CD-ROM icons ie ➡. These icons flag up additional information related to a topic that can be found on the CD-ROM.

Computer compatibility and how to use the CD-ROM

The CD-ROM contains a series of Word, Powerpoint and PDF documents which are viewed though a web browser (either Internet Explorer or Netscape Navigator). Please note that you will need one of these browsers installed on your machine before you can access the contents of this CD-ROM.

Hardware

To use the CD-ROM you must have a Windows PC 486 or higher with a CD-ROM drive. Most of the material is contained on the CD-ROM itself. However, there are also some links to useful Internet sites. To take advantage of this tool, you must have an Internet connection.

Software

To view the documents, you must have the following software installed on your computer:

- Internet Explorer v. 2 or higher or Netscape Navigator v. 2.0 or higher.
  (If you have any of this software already installed on your computer, but would like to upgrade, simply follow the links on the CD-ROM to the web sites where you will be able to download the upgraded software free of charge.)

- Microsoft Word 6.0 or higher.

- Microsoft Excel 5.1 or higher.

Using the CD-ROM

If your PC meets all the hardware and software requirements:

- Insert the CD-ROM in the CD drive and close. The CD-ROM should automatically launch your web browser, and open the CD-ROM.
- If the web browser does not automatically launch, open your web browser (either Internet Explorer or Netscape Navigator).
- Choose File – Open – Browse and select Index.htm from the D or E drive of your PC.
- From here you can navigate the site by clicking on the links that appear.

To install the contents of the CD-ROM to your hard drive:

- Create a folder in c:/
- Give the folder a name you will associate with the CD-ROM eg HSJCD
- Copy the entire contents of the CD-ROM
- Paste into c:/HSJCD.

Using template documents

You can open a Word document by clicking on the title of the document as it appears in your browser. When the document has opened, save it to your hard drive (C directory). You will then be able to make changes to the document and print.

Appendix B – Response to the *Kennedy Report*

The NHS Leadership Centre's response to the *Kennedy Report*	
Recommendation	**Action**
The centre, along with trusts, should develop training and support programmes for clinicians and others seeking to become executive directors.	Our executive director development programme begins in January 2002 with a strong multi-professional approach. We can apply the lessons to help trusts design local programmes.
Newly appointed non-executive directors of health organisations should receive an induction programme including NHS values and responsibilities about the quality of care.	We are working with regional appointments commissioners on an induction guide for non-executives to be available in early 2002.
Non-executive directors should have training support and advice organised through the NHS Leadership Centre.	We are working with regional commissioners on development programmes for non-executive directors. We are building on some excellent regional work and will design a menu of activity to support chairs and non-executive directors.
Chairs of trust boards should have independent advice or a mentor drawn from a pool of experts assembled by the NHS Leadership Centre.	We have a huge amount of knowledge about people with the skills and expertise to mentor chairs. We will be the broker to bring people together.
The NHS Leadership Centre should offer guidelines on acceptable and unacceptable leadership styles and practices in the NHS.	We are developing a set of measurable standards on leadership values and behaviours. This can be used to select, appraise and develop leaders at all levels of the NHS.
People with the potential to lead within the NHS should be identified and trained. There should be sustained investment in developing leadership skills at all levels in the NHS.	We will distribute values and behaviours standards across the NHS so that local programmes are consistent. We are making a large investment in leadership development for chief executives, nurses and executive directors, including mentoring and coaching. Our management training scheme – MTS – for graduates is a key part of our investment in future leaders.

Recommendation	Action
NHS programmes on leadership skills should focus on joint education and multi-professional training open to nurses, doctors, managers and other healthcare professionals.	Our new executive director development programme focuses on the multi-professional roles and responsibilities for medical and nursing directors and their work with general and financial managers.
The NHS Leadership Centre should be involved in all stages of the education, training and continuing development of all healthcare professionals.	We work alongside colleagues from workforce development confederations and higher education to influence curriculum planning and will be supporting the development of the new NHS University.
Any clinician, before appointment to a managerial role must demonstrate they are competent to take on the new role and should get training and support from their organisation.	Our clinical director and medical director development programmes began in Autumn 2001 and include lessons from Bristol. There is a strong emphasis on the skills needed to lead and manage change. We will share our ideas and learn from good practice in local health organisations.
Clinicians should not be required or expected to hold managerial roles on any basis other than competence for the job.	The standards in our values and behaviours framework will apply in these situations and will help to minimise the scope for inappropriate appointments.
The involvement of the public, particularly of patients should not be limited to the representatives of patient groups, or to those representing the interests of patients with a particular illness or condition.	We have done a study that shows how closely leadership behaviour is linked to the patient experience. We have started a national citizen leadership programme that supports patients' representatives in developing a leadership role and aims to develop leadership skills to support self-care and 'expert patients'.

Appendix C — Answer to the 9 dots puzzle

One solution to the thinking outside the box
puzzle on page 111 is shown below. 111

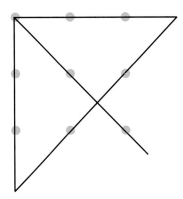

Notes